Healing Cancer With Common Sense

The Official Workbook To The Bestselling Documentary "CANCER is curable NOW"

D1551661

By Marcus & Sabrina Freudenmann

Healing Cancer With Common Sense

The Official Workbook To The Bestselling Documentary
"CANCER is curable NOW"

by Marcus & Sabrina Freudenmann

Published March 2012

Printed in USA by Bang Printing Brainerd, MN

ISBN: 978-0-9870869-1-4

Contents

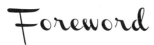

Foreword

Cancer is marketed as INCURABLE.

If you claim there's a cure you unleash a storm of nasty letters and legal prosecution to shut you up.

But despite this effort to suppress the truth lots of people are healing cancer permanently.

<u>**This workbook shows you how they do it.**</u>

For nearly a hundred years, we've all been led to believe that the modern-day medical establishment has thrown the kitchen sink at various forms of cancer.

So why has it achieved only anemic, lackluster results to date?

Because throwing a kitchen sink at patients usually crushes or kills them!

After watching loved ones die slow, ghastly deaths induced by the side effects of chemo or radiation, it occurred to us to ask the right question: Does it make sense to use toxic chemicals and harmful radiation into bodies that are already critically taxed?

We knew intuitively—as does anyone who ponders this question logically—that there had to be better ways to heal cancer. So we went in search of them.

Did we find THE cure for cancer? **No.**

Did we find people who have legitimately and permanently healed cancer to live out the rest of their lives cancer-free? **Yes.**

Did we find alternative clinical settings that avoid contemporary chemotherapy and radiation while employing more logical, sensible, COMMON SENSE solutions that work more often than do conventional methods? **Yes.**

Our journey

After a dear friend was killed by the side effects of a radical course of chemotherapy just a week before her first grandchild was born, we were sick with anger toward the oncologist who had insisted on the treatment. Our dear friend had considered his wisdom second only to God's. She fully believed what he was telling her. Based on her trust in medical science we couldn't convince her otherwise. Even if she'd done nothing instead of the aggressive chemo, we're certain she would have lived to enjoy the pleasure of holding her first grandchild in her arms and watching him grow.

After seeing James and Laurentine's documentary FOOD MATTERS we were inspired to follow in their footsteps; to travel the world and discover all we could about healing cancer holistically. We decided we'd make a movie along the way, filled with interviews and insights, and share everything we learned with people fighting cancer (and their loved ones).

We sold everything we had (home, horses, dogs, clinic, office, car, business, and everything else), packed up the kids, and began the greatest adventure of our lives.

We planned a year-long voyage of discovery. Little did we know it would grow to nearly three years in length!

During our journey, we interviewed scores of long-term cancer survivors, asking them what they did and what kinds of treatment they'd used to overcome the scourges that had invaded their bodies. These candid, eye-opening, one-on-one interviews led us to the clinics and physicians these long-term survivors had consulted and relied on to achieve the results they got.

We visited more than 150 clinics, doctors, scientists and long term survivors, staying with each of them for several days or weeks. We watched the treatment protocols, the lifestyle changes; we spoke with patients to gain an incredible overview of what works and what doesn't.

Sadly, many of the clinics we visited were half-hearted, focusing solely on one or two specialty treatments while leaving out many of the fundamental details. For example, the "hospital food" in some clinics was horrendous, despite the doctors' thirty-minute lecture on how vital proper diet is to the recovery of wellbeing. In fact their dietary programs destroyed all the other proactive efforts to help the patient. These clinics had significantly less success and didn't vary much from the conventional approach: reducing tumor size at all costs but **without** addressing the cause to help heal and protect the patient from recurrence.

It was clinics and practitioners like the ones in the paragraph above that give the oncology profession its dreary reputation.

But there were practitioners in other places who worked on reducing the tumor, while giving their patients life-saving education, cooking classes and other methods to change unhealthy behaviors and give their patients' immune systems the boost they needed to detoxify and offer better outcomes.

Many things cause illness and weaken the immune system. Clinics, doctors and naturopaths who address the **CAUSE** while helping the body heal, are clearly leading the battle against cancer and other illnesses.

We witnessed something else, too: Most of the patients who were willing to change the things that had fostered their ill health achieved better results than those who were unwilling to make changes.

The best results happened for patients who invested whole-heartedly in a healthy lifestyle, a healthy diet, and other methods of re-booting their immune systems. They detoxified regularly and diligently, taking slow-but-steady steps to rebuild their lives. Some sold their businesses, dropped out of toxic relationships, and stopped doing everything else that thwarted their spirits. Many of them began to travel, make music, and invest in whatever filled their hearts with true joy and meaning.

At its essence, to be healthy means to thwart disease and illness.

Our journey massively changed our own lifestyles, diets and day-to-day choices. We believe it was the greatest education our children will ever receive and we are grateful to be able to share what we have learned with you.

At journey's end, we were in Canada with more than 200 hours of HD video footage from twelve different countries. That's when the truly-tedious work began. It took nine months just to edit the videos.

We prepared ninety seven folders, one for every subject (detoxification, supplementation, toxins, treatments, etc.). Each of the interviews was then cut and clips went into their proper folder.

While listening a second (sometimes a third and fourth) time to the videotaped doctors, we recognized additional nuggets of wisdom we hadn't "caught" before. As it turns out, the human mind has to **open** to a subject first; only then can it discern the finest strains within the orchestra.

After we filled the folders, we created the storyline and cut the first draft to about 8 hours in length.

During the next two months I deleted redundancies and anything else I considered of minor import, managing in the process to reduce the movie to four hours. Then, with scalpel-like precision, I removed all but 110 minutes of video. It was a painful process, but viewers are accustomed to watching videos of two hours or less, and I wanted to honor the custom.

After the movie debuted, I planned to use the unused clips (mostly interviews with cancer survivors) for another movie, but as Sabrina began to write a compilation of all the treatments for a workshop we quickly understood that a workbook can guide patients just as well as—if not better than—a movie. With a workbook before you, you can take all the time you need to discover what you need to do to heal cancer yourself.

You're holding the result in your hands. It has been a true labor of love and we believe it will help you.

Due to the problems we had, as outlined in the title of this foreword, we've chosen a different title for the workbook. We're calling it **Healing Cancer with Common Sense**.

If you will apply common sense to the challenge, you will understand the significance and truth we've collected here. It's not about proof and results (proof and results have been faked by moneyed interests time after time; you read the news regularly, we presume.); it's about **common sense**. Simply employ your common sense as you work your way through our workbook and you'll be amazed by what jumps out at you!

One last thing: We never try to convince anyone of anything. If this approach is not for you, we fully respect your right to ignore it. Everyone has a different path and lesson to learn; there is no right or wrong choice. There is just **your** choice. All we offer is what we've discovered while learning from those who have traveled the path before you. That's what we're sharing with you.

With love,

Marcus and Sabrina Freudenmann

About the Authors

German-born Sabrina Freudenmann ND has invested years of research and a lifetime of study in the holistic treatment of degenerative diseases. She is also an Ayurvedic practitioner and has studied Anthroposophical lifestyle science. Her passion for the subject makes her an expert in pursuing the cause of diseases and recommending solutions that reveal great promise in eliminating or alleviating them.

Sabrina is dedicated to changing the world through teaching and writing and by living the change she wants to see in the world. She has given birth to all four children at home. She has developed her own curriculum and home schools all four children. As co-producer of the movie Sabrina also studies and researches the topic endlessly. She is the co-author of this workbook. Her speed, efficiency and accuracy in research are extraordinary.

Marcus Freudenmann holds a Masters in architecture and interior design. He also has diplomas in art, graphic design and computer visualization. As an entrepreneur with a sense for adventure, Marcus has enjoyed great success in Germany. His success has allowed him to live a life of luxury. When their first son Benedict was born in 1992 with severe skin eczema, Marcus and Sabrina discovered that it's not money that makes them happy but a healthy relationship and a healthy body. This instigated their move to New Zealand and Australia where they started a new life dedicated to alert consciousness for nature and the human body, mind and spirit.

Marcus has since shifted his focus to his real passion: philosophy, spirituality and psychology. He's become an accomplished scholar of Vedantic scriptures and the Mahayana sutras and has works with clients to help them discover their "blessings in disguise". His workshops, "Loving Cancer" and "Love Your problems", has been downloaded more than 15,000 times. His studies and work with clients have made Marcus an expert in Emotional Intelligence which he now teaches at the EQ ACADEMY.

Marcus is the producer of the movie CANCER is curable NOW which you can find at www.CancerIsCurableNow.tv and has a free online resource for cancer patients at www.maxawareness.com

Acknowledgements

We want to express our gratitude to all of the doctors, naturopaths, and health practitioners with years of experience who shared their wisdom in our newsletters and who spent hours and days explaining, recording, and showing us the most relevant basics of life for our movie. We would not be able to present this workbook to you without their knowledge and participation.

I would also like to include Dr. Mercola, Mike Adams, Dr. Mark Hyman, Mark Sircus, Dr. Keith Scott Mumby, Dr. Josh Axe, and Ken Cook from the EWG, and many more. These educators have been our constant companions for years, and their efforts in sharing valuable insights are highly admirable. Dr. Epstein, from Cancer Prevention has also been our partner for many years. We don't know where we would be without them. I am also eternally grateful to Dr. John F. Demartini who inspired me to see and understand Emotional Intelligence. It's what has changed my life so incredibly, and I am happy to share it with you.

There are lights before us and there will be lights after us, but only if we freely share what we have learned. In this way we can brighten the world. And that's what we would like to ask you to do as a very first step in your journey through this book.

WHO IS YOUR STUDENT?

Please write below a list of people with whom you would like to share what you learn in this book:

_____

_____

_____

_____

_____

Disclaimer

The information in this "Healing Cancer With Common Sense" Workbook and the Movie "CANCER is curable NOW," as well as the Director's Cut of CICN is intended for informational purposes only. Marcus and Sabrina Freudenmann (the Authors) as well as maxAwareness Pty. Ltd. are not responsible for your decisions resulting from the use of the information, including, but not limited to, your choosing to seek or not to seek professional medical care, or from choosing or not choosing specific treatment based on the information.

Marcus and Sabrina Freudenmann (the Authors) as well as maxAwareness Pty. Ltd. encourage persons who wish to embark on a health or treatment program to contact and be supervised by a qualified health care practitioner. We do, though, recommend to not take simply the nearest and first best doctor, but rather search for a partner who really has a track record of helping patients to get well.

The workbook "Healing Cancer With Common Sense," as well as the movie, contain information including data, statistics, and research from third parties.

Marcus and Sabrina Freudenmann (the Authors), as well as MaxAwareness Pty. Ltd., and any other person involved in the making and distribution of the workbook and film do not warrant the accuracy, reliability, currency, or completeness of those views or statements presented in the movie and workbook and do not assume or accept any legal liability whatsoever for the accuracy, quality, suitability, and currency of the information and the subject matter of the film and workbook.

Views and statements expressed in the film and workbook are not substitutes for independent professional advice. Viewers should exercise their own care, skill, and diligence with respect to the reliance and use of any information contained in the film and workbook. Viewers should not act or refrain from acting on information in the film and workbook without first taking appropriate professional advice in respect of their own particular circumstances.

The content found here is for informational purposes only and is in no way intended as medical advice, as a substitute for medical counseling, or as a treatment/cure for any disease or health condition, nor should it be construed as such. Always work with a qualified health professional before making any changes to your diet, prescription drug use, lifestyle, or exercise activities. This information is provided as-is, and the reader/viewer assumes all risks from the use, non-use, or misuse of this information.

State Your Purpose

The second thing we would like you to do, even before you start, is to declare your purpose.

Our mind is programmed to see and understand what we focus on. If you walk through a shopping center with a clear image of what you are looking for, you are most likely to find it or see that it's not there. Your mind will process every possible opportunity to fulfill the purpose. That's why it's crucial that you know what you want to gain from this book in order to find it.

What do you want to gain

- **from this workshop,**
- **from reading this workbook,**
- **from watching this workshop DVD?**

State very clearly the outcome you envision. The more detailed and accurate you declare the purpose, the more likely it is you will achieve it.

_____

_____

_____

_____

_____

_____

_____

_____

What Is Cancer?

Mainstream doctors, pharmaceutical companies, and the media have demonized cancer as YOUR ENEMY. Let's go to war against cancer, and let's fight this horrible disease. Cancer is bad, dark, painful, and horrible, and it can come to everybody with only one purpose: TO KILL!

They will tell you that, so far, we have not found an effective weapon against this terrifying disease, but, if you give us more money, we might be able to find a solution soon. In fact, we are close. The new drug is just around the corner. We just need another couple of billion $$$$$ to solve the mystery.

☯ CANCER IS NOT YOUR ENEMY.

As a matter of fact, cancer is your friend. It's a wakeup call. It's what we all need in order to grow, evolve, and learn. Many have called cancer an OPPORTUNITY to grow beyond their present limitations. Others have called cancer a STOP sign that indicates to us that we are heading in the wrong direction.

Cancer helps you find the motivation for change. It's your driving force to a much better life. Without it, you would probably continue your miserable life and not even know that you could feel much better. Most people are so used to their aches and pains that they can't remember life without them.

Cancer helps you to reconnect with who you truly are. It also helps you to connect with much deeper parts of yourself that you might have forgotten about. Spirituality, passion, presence, and awareness are always a result of this friend knocking on your door.

Cancer also helps save this world from abuse, rape, and destruction. Without the growing number of cancer cases, mankind would never wake up to the fact that our lifestyle is actually killing the planet and everything that lives on it. Again, it's a friend who points out that we are on the wrong path—a path of destruction.

☯ CANCER IS A SYMPTOM

When you drive your car and the warning light comes on, you do not smash the red light and keep going. You react to the warning and look for the cause. This is what we call common sense.

You search for the reason that the light came on because it means there is a problem.

Possible reasons that the warning light for your health came on can be:

Deficiencies.

You are low in oils, minerals, vitamins, essential fatty acids, etc.

Blocked / Dirt / Toxic.

If your air filter is blocked, you don't get enough oxygen, and your engine will not run properly.

If your blood filters are clogged up, you can't filter out all the toxins, so the whole system breaks down.

If your exhaust is blocked, you can't get rid of toxic waste, which poisons you from the inside out.

Bad Fuel.

You have filled your engine with bad or inadequate food, and your engine is not running on max power—or perhaps it's not running at all!

Stiff and Cranky

Your tires are flat, your joints and bearings are without any lubrication, and it's painful to move. Therefore, you'd rather move less so that it does not hurt.

Low battery

Your batteries are exhausted from the constant overload. You pull more voltage than you recharge. You install too many high voltage gadgets and toys and wonder why all your fuses pop.

There are probably a few more problems which could be listed, such as the clutter you keep in your car and the attitude of the driver who is in a terrible mood, but I think you get the picture. Cancer is not the problem in the first place. It grows because you have other problems, which cause the red lights to come on and the sirens to alarm.

You Are Unique

This is a very critical point in healing.

We are all different and unique and there is no single protocol that fits all of us. Yes, there are commonalities, and a detox is probably good for everyone. But there are many things that can poison you that might need to be detoxed from your system depending on your environment and your problems. You might have mercury-related problems, or maybe you are full of phthalates and other cosmetic toxins. Deficiencies are also a common problem, but what you are deficient in differs from person to person.

In order to truly heal, you need to take into account all aspects of your life. Dr. Leigh Erin Connealy, David Getoff, and all of the others doctors we feature in the movie do this. They check into hundreds of factors which can lead to the disease in the first place.

The difference between you and anyone else starts with your genes.

- Did you inherit a solid, strong immune system or a weak one?

- Did you get a high toxic load from your mother?

- Are you from healthy stock, or do all of your ancestors suffer from certain deficiencies and diseases?

- Have your parents lived a health-conscious life and maintained a healthy environment at home, or did no one care?

- Right from the start, did you get a big load of toxins with all the vaccines they injected into your young body, or did your parents refrain from getting you these toxic vaccinations?

- Did you get loads of antibiotics (anti-life) at a young age, destroying your natural immune system and intestinal milieu?

- Did you grow up walking in plenty of fresh air and playing sports, or did you grow up in a concrete jungle with high pollution and daily video game and TV sessions?

- Did you grow up on a farm with plenty of toxins, fertilizers, sprays, antibiotics, and other toxins?

- Did you . . . As you can see already in those seven questions, you have a huge variety of possibilities, and the list could be 100 questions long. That's why it's essential that your health practitioner regards you as an individual and designs a treatment program suited to your needs.

We are a whole, living being, and there is no separation between our mind and physical body. That's why it's crucial to understand your mental and emotional composure. Your mental attitude and your passion for life are of the utmost importance. If you have heavy emotional burdens that pull you down and you see disease as a blessing because it frees you from your daily routine, then all the healing in the world cannot help you. If your partner finally looks after you just because you are sick, when he or she never cared before, it's going to be hard to get you well because you might fear that your relationship will return to its old status.

Another really important part is that no organ operates by itself; everything is linked and interwoven with each other. Consequently, a weak thyroid or any other organ can create a chain reaction that eventually leads to a more serious condition like cancer. But in a case like that, it's very hard to determine the original source of the problem. It could be a hereditary factor; therefore, it might be necessary to include your family history into the diagnosis.

There are hundreds of different combinations and pathways which lead to cancer; therefore, every cancer protocol needs to be fitted personally to you.

What is right for you can be wrong for someone else.

While you are reading and working through this book, we want you to highlight everything that you feel is relevant for your recovery with a yellow marker. This way you can come back later and understand perfectly what needs to be changed in order to get well.

Don't forget that disease is a process and never appears out of the blue without warning. We have many warning signs and symptoms before any kind of disease actually develops. Cancer is one of the last stages of a body's breakdown. Many other imbalances and diseases were apparent beforehand.

As disease is a process, healing is a process too. You cannot expect to be healed in a month or maybe even a year. Your body needs time to heal and mend. No chronic disease can be turned around instantaneously or speedily. You may feel an improvement in a very short time, but you must not stop there because the true healing has just begun.

Life is a process, disease is a process and cure is a process.

CHAPTER 1

Find The Cause And Remove It

☯ CERTAIN THINGS CAUSE CANCER.

Is that really so?

- Some people smoke for years without getting cancer, while others get cancer even though they never smoked their whole life.

- Some eat an unhealthy diet and remain well, while others get sick even though they eat a healthy, organic diet for years.

- Some spend much of their time out in the sun and never have a spot of skin cancer, while others have it in areas that aren't even exposed to the sun.

The problem is that mankind tries to simplify things without understanding the big picture. They pathologies the problem, give it a name, and then try to eradicate it. They want to blame their problem on an outside cause.

There are hundreds of research papers that blame VIRUSES or INFLAMMATIONS, GENES or INFECTIONS, TOXINS or CARCINOGENS for causing cancer. I believe they are going to find more and more cancer-causing agents because it allows them to develop and market a variety of new weapons/drugs to be used in the war against the disease. The more problems and causes they find, the more drugs they can prescribe, and the more money they can earn.

But they never look at the real problem—THE CAUSE.

☯ OUR IMMUNE SYSTEM CAN'T COPE WITH THE BURDEN!

The reason you get sick is that you overload your immune system. Your body is designed to handle many challenges at the same time, but if the load becomes too much or there are too many battles being fought at the same time, your immune system collapses and disease sets in.

- There are over 80,000 TOXINS in our environment.

- There are over 14,000 known and proven CARCINOGENS in our food, water, and environment.
- There are over 12 million different VIRUSES.
- There are over 19 million FUNGI and BACTERIA.
- There are countless problems caused by DEFICIENCIES.
- There are numerous INFLAMMATIONS and INFECTIONS.
- Plus, there is **your** LIFESTYLE!

LIFESTYLE CHOICES either **support** or **challenge** your immune system. It's as simple as that.

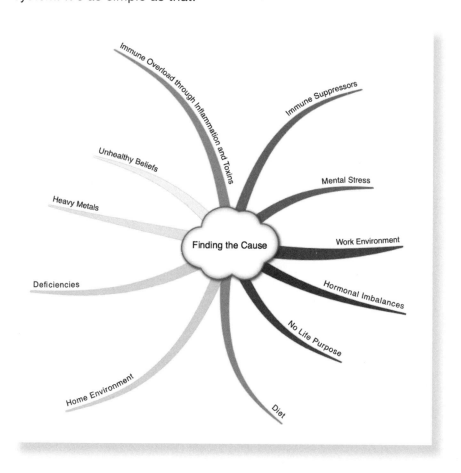

Physical Causes

Never ever think that you got cancer or any other degenerative disease because someone coughed on you. It was not some strange accident over which you had no control. It's a disease that persists over many years and only develops because your immune system is not able to keep up with the job.

Imagine your immune system as an army of white blood cells. These cells are willing and able to defend your body, but only if they are strong, well trained, well rested, and well fed.

What if these cells are not well trained? What if they are lazy and fat? What if they have been fed loads of food that they are not supposed to eat and very little food high in nutritional value? What if they have little to no oxygen? What if they live in a messy environment and their living conditions are absolutely debilitating?

Do you think they can adequately defend you from all the dangers? Would you trust such an army to keep you safe?

Immune Suppressors

In this first list, we talk about things that kill or immobilize your immune system!

☯ SUGAR

It's hard to believe that sugar is the #1 killer in the world. And we are all addicted to it. It's like a gun that fires in slow-motion, and you happily place it in your mouth and pull the trigger.

If you feed sugar to the soldiers of your defense army, it's like giving them a sleeping pill. They will be out of service for one to four hours. How can you expect them to be on the front-line defending your body with a fat belly and in the mood for a nap?

It doesn't make sense that you sedate the soldiers prior to sending them off to the battlefield and then expect them to adequately protect and defend your body!

If your breakfast consists of hot chocolate, cereal, and some donuts, your body is already running on sugar overload first thing in the morning. All of these carbohydrates are immediately converted into sugar and knock your immune system out until lunch.

Then you have a sandwich, or, because it smells so good, some macaroni and cheese followed by dessert. WOW! Now your immune soldiers can rest until dinner. Imagine those guys lying around with big fat bellies and no energy to do anything.

> *It is common sense that you have to remove the cause first in order to stop the problem. As soon as you remove the cause, everything will automatically get better.* --- Bill Henderson

Then as your workday finally comes to an end, you go home and have a bottle or two of beer and possibly an extra large pizza followed by some chips or cookies as you settle in for the night with a good bottle of wine or a rum and Coke. That should disable your immune system until morning when you can begin your day with more sedatives. We forgot to mention the five sodas you had in between your meals—they alone can suppress your immune response for days.

And while your immune system is completely inactive, your cancer cells are thriving on this sugar consumption. They gobble it all up, and they explode with energy and growth.

Sugar has a double whammy effect. It disables, disrupts, and distracts your immune system, but it also reactivates, re-energizes, and replenishes your cancer cells, which enables them to grow at a greater, faster, and stronger rate.

What Makes Sugar so Appealing to Cancer Cells?

In 1931 the Nobel Prize was awarded to a German researcher, Dr. Otto Warburg, who first discovered that cancer cells have a fundamentally different energy metabolism compared to healthy cells. Malignant tumors tend to use glucose as fuel for the cancer cells, creating lactic acid as a byproduct. The large amount of lactic acid produced by this fermentation of glucose from cancer cells is then transported to your liver.

This conversion of glucose to lactic acid generates a lower, more acidic pH in cancerous tissues as well as an overall physical fatigue from lactic acid buildup.

This is a very inefficient pathway for energy metabolism, as it extracts only about 5 percent of the available energy from your food supply. In simplistic terms, the cancer is "wasting" energy, which causes you to become both tired and undernourished.

In addition, the carbohydrates from glucose and sucrose will significantly decrease the capacity of neutrophils to do their job. Neutrophils are a type of white blood cell that help cells to envelope and destroy invaders, such as cancer. Meanwhile, fructose appears to be preferred by cancer cells for cell division, which contributes to its growth and to its spreading throughout your body.

Even though the theory that sugar feeds cancer was born nearly 80 years ago, most conventional cancer programs STILL do not adequately address diet and the need to avoid sugars and fructose if you have cancer.

As Patrick Quillin, PhD, RD, CNS wrote more than a decade ago:

> *"During the last 10 years I have worked with more than 500 cancer patients as director of nutrition for Cancer Treatment Centers of America in Tulsa, Okla. It puzzles me why the simple concept 'sugar feeds cancer' can be so dramatically overlooked as part of a comprehensive cancer treatment plan. Of the millions of cancer patients being treated in America today, hardly any are offered any scientifically guided nutrition therapy beyond being told to 'just eat good foods.' Most patients I work with arrive with a complete lack of nutritional advice."*

(http://articles.mercola.com/sites/articles/archive/2011/09/29/is-this-simple-sugar-a-major-factor-in-th-failure-of-the-war-on-cancer.aspx)

☯ ACIDITY

Imagine that you have to work in an acidic environment. Your skin burns, your eyes water, you can hardly breathe, and you are drained of all energy. You are half paralyzed with blurry vision, and everything you do is doubly exhausting.

This is how your army of defense and all your cells feel in an acidic body. Acidity is caused by the cancer itself, by lack of exercise, and by an uneducated diet filled with loads of denatured proteins / fatty meats which have been processed and cooked, hydrogenated fats, artificial sweeteners, chocolates, peanuts, wheat, white flour, pastries, pastas, cheese, homogenized milk, ice cream, beer, soft drinks, plus loads of coffee and sugar in any given form. With this kind of diet, every single cell in your body runs at only 20 to 30 percent of its capacity.

And don't think your brain is spared when we talk about acidity. In fact, it's one of the first things to suffer from high acidity. You can't think clearly, and your mind is dulled.

Acidity is the breeding ground for cancer cells. Every cell will degenerate and become sick when it is in an acidic environment too long. When dividing into new cells, they create sick, weird, abnormal, and cancerous cells.

CANCER THRIVES IN AN ACIDIC ENVIRONMENT

☯ LOW OXYGEN ENVIRONMENT

Low oxygenation in your body is called an anaerobic living space that causes your cancer cells to thrive while your healthy cells die.

Just stop breathing oxygen for a moment (not too long please). That's how your army of defense feels in an anaerobic body.

No one can live without oxygen and neither can your white blood cells. If there is not enough oxygen, they either die, or they just hang around, barely surviving. Not only does a lack of oxygen make them weak and exhausted, but your immune cells need oxygen to have the killing effect they need to destroy cancer cells.

Cancer cells, on the other hand, have learned to live without oxygen. They don't need oxygen to survive. In fact, they actually hate it because an anaerobic environment is the perfect living space for them.

Therefore, lack of oxygen also has a double whammy effect because the anaerobic environment protects the cancer and your army of defense can't reach the tumor without being completely exhausted.

Dr. Warburg proposed that normalizing the metabolism of cancer cells was the key to effective cancer treatment, and the means to accomplish this was to increase the oxygen content of the cells.

> *Dr. Warburg stated that as the first priority of treatment, "-- all growing body cells be saturated with oxygen," and the second priority was to avoid further exposure to toxins.*

☯ LITTLE TO NO SLEEP

Your body detoxifies and regenerates during sleep; this is when it actually heals itself. That's why when children get sick, they go to bed and sleep it off. It's the natural healing reaction of the body.

If your body doesn't get enough of this healing time, you slowly exhaust all of your reserves to the point where the body can't heal any more.

Hormones are a huge part of the healing effects of sleep. During deep sleep, your body produces the growth hormone at its maximum level. Growth hormones speed up the absorption of nutrients and amino acids into your cells and aid in the healing of tissues throughout your body. Hormones also stimulate your bone marrow, where your immune cells are born.

Melatonin, often called the sleep hormone, is also produced during sleep. This hormone inhibits tumors from growing, prevents viral infections, stimulates your immune system, increases antibodies in your saliva, has antioxidant properties, and enhances the quality of sleep.

One of the most commonly described effects of a cancer diagnosis is the deprivation of sleep due to fear, stress, and worry. This side effect alone will cost you weeks and even months of your life.

Therefore, it is essential to do whatever is necessary to get adequate sleep. And we aren't talking about sleeping pills, which also put your healing mechanism to sleep. We are referring to methods that make you tired, relax the mind, and help you to fall into a deep, healing sleep.

Here are a few tips that can help you to sleep better:

- Try to sleep in complete darkness and block out any light that comes from the outside or from light sources like your clock radio in your bedroom. Light hinders the production of melatonin and serotonin, which are needed for a speedy recovery.
- Keep your bedroom free of clutter and reserve it for sleeping only.

Ventilate the room and sleep with open windows whenever possible.

A cool temperature will also help you sleep.

Check your bedroom for EMFs (electromagnetic fields). These fields can disrupt the production of melatonin and stress your organisms.

Try to wind down before you go to sleep. Do not watch scary or emotionally arousing movies. One hour prior to bedtime, your activities should be calming and relaxing.

Exercise will always result in better sleep at night.

Have your magnesium levels checked as sufficient magnesium will calm and relax your whole body. A magnesium bath can work miracles and will transport you into a deep sleep.

Have your adrenals checked by a good, natural medicine physician.

Go to bed early and get up early.

Signs of Sleep Deprivation

- Frequent waking, teeth grinding, snoring, sleep apnoea, nightmares

- Waking up in the morning fatigued
- Poor motivation
- Irritability
- Depression, anxiety
- Headaches
- Tired during day
- Falling asleep while sitting and reading
- Sudden sleep periods
- Comprised immune system
- Increased cravings for sugar, coffee, alcohol, recreational drugs
- Bad concentration

☯ STRESS

While under stress, your body goes into a FIGHT or FLIGHT mode. This is a beneficial mechanism if you are in real danger, but when this stress is prolonged or becomes chronic, this condition has a very adverse effect on your body. The fight or flight response is mediated by the autonomic nervous system which is responsible for TWO other body systems.

The immune system:

- Lymph nodes
- Tonsils
- Adenoids
- Thymus
- Bone marrow
- Spleen
- Mesenteric lymph
- Peyer's Patch

The endocrine system

- Hypothalamus
- Pineal
- Pituitaries
- Parathyrin
- Thyroid
- Thymus
- Stomach
- Adrenal
- Kidney
- Pancreas
- Duodenum
- Uterus
- Ovary
- Testis

Stress causes a great deal of wear and tear on these organs.

Stress can result from many things, and it starts with the "alarm state" caused by fear and anxiety. These signals first stimulate the hypothalamus and then the endocrine and the immune systems, followed by the autonomic nervous system.

The alarm state causes an outpouring of CORTISOL from the adrenal glands, which is the stress hormone of the endocrine system.

At the same time, the shrinking of the lymph nodes and thymus reduces the functionality of the immune system.

The increased Cortisol and insulin levels in the body, accompanied by an increase in blood sugar, lead to a stressed immune response. Combined with high levels of LDL, which are the bad fats in cholesterol, you will experience an increase in your blood pressure, heart rates, and your level of fatigue.

The vicious cycle of diseases relating to this initial stress reaction is endless. Each disease that plagues your body can lead to other conditions or diseases. For instance, irritable bowel syndrome also leads to leaky gut and infectious diseases of the intestines, which, in turn, lead to poor absorption, deficiencies, and the re-absorption of toxins. This snowball effect occurs in nearly every disease our body encounters.

Stress is a culprit with many ways to express itself in your body and will settle in your weakest organs.

❧ NO EXERCISE

It's a matter of common sense that anything that becomes stagnant has a high likelihood of developing an unfavorable condition. A pond with no circulation will produce a foul odor and fermentation of scum on the surface of the water. This is also how your body responds to the lack of exercise.

The only way to get toxins and dead cells out of your system is through the circulation of body fluids, which are pushed by your heart and by the movement of your muscles.

Blood is the body's main transportation system. It carries oxygen and nutrients to your cells and removes the garbage from your system.

If this process is not functioning sufficiently, then these dead cells, toxins, and waste materials start to accumulate in certain areas of your body and pollute the system. Similar to a landfill or dump, if our garbage is not disposed of properly it will produce toxic gases, foul fluids, and a high level of acidity; it will invite the growth of parasites, bacteria, and fungi. Plus, the surrounding areas suffer huge distress in the form of inflammations.

Due to bad circulation, these dumping sites are not isolated to only one place in your body but develop in several different areas. This causes yet another simultaneous battle for your already starved and paralyzed immune system to fight. Your cells not only lack the nourishment they need to perform their duties, but they are also overwhelmed by an insurmountable and impossible workload. Furthermore, the pathways (blood) used to get to and from work are sluggish and slow and offer hardly any air to breathe.

Can you visualize these conditions?

SOLUTION:

No sugar, loads of greens, plenty of fresh air, good and sound sleep, less stress and more joy, and at least 30 minutes of exercise each day.

Your immune system will love you for it.

Immune Overload

Even under the worst working conditions, your immune system is loyal and dutiful. These little white blood cells love you and do everything they possibly can to defend your body and clean up the mess. However, sometimes they just can't cope with the massive amount of work to be done, or maybe there simply aren't enough of them to do the job.

Again, think of each of the following diseases as the enemy—an enemy which requires thousands of soldiers to defend us against the attack. Depending on the number of enemies you have to battle, you might not have enough soldiers to win the war.

Use Common Sense:

Inflammation is actually a good thing. It is our body's natural response to fight infections and heal trauma. It causes the blood supply to increase so that the body can send building materials and repair troops to the infected area, which are followed by clean-up troops that remove and dispose of all the damaged cells. It's a very busy workplace where increased heat widens the path to avoid a traffic jam, thereby speeding up the healing process.

The problems arise when our immune system gets out of balance and starts to destroy its own kind. In other words, misinformation from the neurotoxins along with deficiencies can lead to chaos.

This will result in conditions like asthma, rheumatoid arthritis, autoimmune disease, and allergies. Hidden inflammations lead to heart disease, obesity, diabetes, dementia, depression, cancer, and even autism. This chronic inflammation destroys our organs and the ability of our cells to function properly.

It is very important to find the cause of these chronic inflammations:

- Poor diet—sugar, refined flours, processed foods, and inflammatory fats such as trans and saturated fats (can lead to leaky gut)

- Food allergies—gluten lactose intolerance (leaky gut)
- Toxins
- Cigarette smoke
- Stress
- Parasites and chronic infections with viruses (i.e. Lyme disease), bacteria (i.e.Campylobacter pylori), or yeasts (Candida)
- Lack of exercise
- Mold toxins and environmental allergens

How do you find out if you have hidden inflammations in your body?

- C-reactive protein in a blood test will give you the degree of hidden inflammation in your body. It is present in all deep-seated, long-term inflammation.
- Interleukin-6 is another hidden inflammation marker as it plays an important role in many chronic inflammatory diseases.

What can you do to eliminate chronic inflammation?

- Get rid of allergens and toxins.
- Detoxify your body of toxins.
- Stop smoking.
- Eat a healthy, whole food diet with healthy fats and **without sugar.**
- Heal your gut with probiotics, multivitamins, omega 3, vitamin D.Exercise regularly.
- Reduce stress.

Inflammatory Diseases

EVERY disease will result in inflammations in your body. It's how your body tries to speed up the repair mechanism. That's why the following list certainly doesn't cover all possible reasons for inflammation, but it will provide you with guidelines to help you in your search for the cause of your disease.

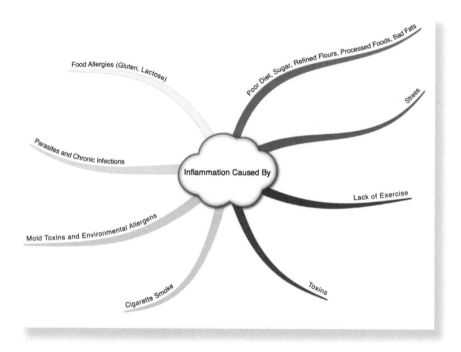

☯ ARTHRITIS

Arthritis literally means inflammation of the joints and is a perfect example of a front-line battle. Inflammation is the body's response to injuries, infections, and deficiencies.

A series of complicated events work to defend the body. Heat and increased blood flow deliver huge numbers of white blood cells to the damaged area that engulf and consume foreign material, dead cartilage, and waste materials for the purpose of tissue repair. For years, these inflammations are a constant battlefield where a war is raging.

☯ LEAKY GUT

"Leaky gut" is a term used to describe a defect in or damage to the inner lining of the intestinal tract, making it less able to filter nutrients and other biological substances needed by the body.

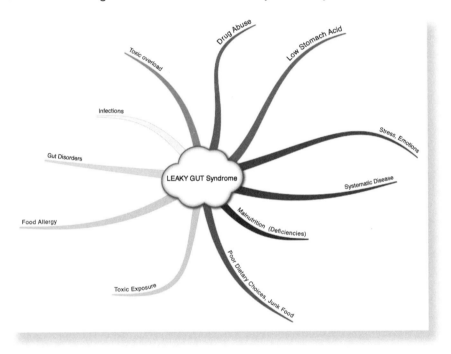

As a consequence, bacteria and other toxins, as well as incompletely digested proteins and fats leak out of the intestines into the bloodstream. This triggers an autoimmune reaction which leads to serious intestinal problems, fatigue, food sensitivities, joint pain, skin rashes, and much more.

The result is a great deal of stress on the immune system, the liver, and every other organ or system in the body.

Common causes for leaky gut are Candida, alcohol, stress, allergies, poor diet, nutritional deficiencies, parasites, and medications.

The most common cause, though, is food allergies, which we will discuss separately. Food allergies constantly trigger inflammations and allergic reactions in the mucous membranes, which cause the defect in the first place.

☯ ULCERS

Ulcers are similar to a leaky gut; they are a weakness in the lining of an external or internal surface of the body caused by a break in the skin or mucous membrane that fails to heal.

Bacterial infections, viruses, stress, spicy foods, serious deficiencies, toxins, alcohol, and more can cause this weakness or damage to the lining. They usually occur in the stomach and upper intestine but can also be found in the mouth.

An ulcer is always a huge burden to the immune system and can grow to a dangerous size, which causes a severe fever reaction and a complete breakdown of your defenses.

☯ LYME DISEASE

Lyme disease is a condition that is created by a specific bacterium that is referred to as "Borrelia Burgdorferi." Humans can acquire this disease when a tick carrying the disease bites them.

Lyme disease is an infection that is described in three phases: early localized disease, early disseminated disease, and late disease. In the early phase of the disease, its symptoms are limited to rashes, flu-like symptoms, and common aches and pain. However, autoimmune and neurodegenerative symptoms may be observed in the advanced stages. The greatest discomfort of Lyme disease is known to be caused by arthritic or rheumatologic symptoms.

During the advanced phases of Lyme disease, the infection interferes with several bodily functions, including circulatory or heart functions as well as functions controlled by the nervous system. As the infection progresses, it may start causing inflammation to the joints, which explains the migratory aches and pains observed among patients.

Blood tests can confirm the diagnosis.

☯ ROSS RIVER VIRUS

Ross River virus is a disease spread by mosquitoes and can cause joint inflammation, pain, fatigue, and muscle aches. The joints most commonly affected are the wrists, knees, ankles, and small joints such as fingers or toes. Swollen lymph nodes and a rash appearing on the trunk and limbs are also present.

Here in Australia, the Ross River virus is widely spread, particularly around inland waterways and coastal regions. Severe epidemics can occur after heavy rainfall, floods, and high tides and temperatures.

The best form of prevention is to avoid mosquito-prone areas, especially at dawn and dusk. Fly screens and mosquito nets also help to reduce the risk of contracting the disease.

Blood tests can confirm the diagnosis.

☯ CAMPYLOBACTER PYLORI INFECTION

Campylobacter infections are among the most common bacterial infections in humans. They produce both diarrheal and systemic illnesses. In industrialized regions, enteric Campylobacter infections produce an inflammatory, sometimes bloody, diarrhea or dysentery syndrome.

Campylobacter jejuni is usually the most common cause of community-acquired inflammatory enteritis. In developing regions, the diarrhea may be watery.

Scientific evidence links this infection to the development of bowel and intestinal cancers.

☯ HELICOBACTER PYLORI INFECTION

Although peptic ulcer disease is the most studied disease related to Helico pylori infection, this bacterium is seemingly involved in the pathogenesis of several extragastric diseases, such as mucosa-associated lymphoid tissue lymphomas, coronaritis, gastroesophageal reflux disease, iron deficiency anemia, skin disease, and rheumatologic conditions.

☯ CANDIDA

Candida, a yeast organism, is normally found on the skin, and in the mouth, gut, and other mucus membranes. Antibiotics and a high sugar diet reduce our natural resistance to its overgrowth and result in infection. These types of infections are sometimes referred to as thrush, oral thrush, yeast infection, or fungal infection. The symptoms, however, could be as simple as "brain fog" or simply feeling lethargic.

A disseminated infection of internal organs by Candida can occur in severely immune-compromised patients, such as those with cancer, serious burns, or AIDS. This is a much more serious condition than a superficial Candida infection.

Candida is one of the most common issues we face. Of the world's population, 98 percent has this disease, and it's growing drastically due to our modern diet.

Dr. Simoncini makes the connection that fungal colonies and cancer colonies are the same colonies called by two different names.

Candida is believed to play a part in creating what is called a "leaky gut," an unfavorable increase in intestinal permeability.

Candida infection has been found to produce 79 distinct toxins.

Extreme cases of Candida cause an allergic response from the body, which further plunders the resources of the body's immune system.

☯ MOLD

Mold is considered to be an extremely small and dangerous organism that belongs to the fungi family.

Molds are associated with damp buildings, and the National Institute for Occupational Safety and Health (NIOSH) says that over 50 percent of US buildings are mold-infected.

Mold Illness begins insidiously as it silently takes away energy, cognition, and easy breathing. It leaves behind pain, fatigue, and often weight gain.

The symptoms of mold exposure may not seem life-threatening at the onset, but over time more serious illnesses may develop.

If you are experiencing several of the following symptoms, mold illness could be the cause.

- Nasal congestion
- Fatigue
- Irritation of the eyes
- Weakness of muscles
- Inflammation of sinuses
- Breathlessness
- Headache
- Runny nose
- Cough
- Sore throat
- Hoarseness
- Muscle cramps
- Abdominal pain

- Stiffness
- Mood swings
- Night sweats
- Vertigo
- Numbness
- Tremors
- Confusion
- Concentration issues

Red eyesMold illness is not an allergy but an inflammation within the body that severely stresses the immune system. Mold toxins attach themselves to fat cells within the body, causing them to continuously release inflammatory cytokines. This results in chronic inflammation, which has devastating effects on your health. Reduced circulation in small blood vessels caused by mold exposure results in reduced oxygen levels in the cells, heart disease, nerve damage, and autoimmune disease.

"Toxicological evidence obtained in vivo and in vitro supports these findings, showing the occurrence of diverse inflammatory and toxic responses after exposure to microorganisms isolated from damp buildings, including their spores, metabolites and component." --- The World Health Organization

What to do?

Eliminate the cause! Look for the moisture in your house or apartment. There are many sources of water intrusion commonly seen in both brand new and older construction. Crawl spaces and basements are the biggest offenders. Look for water coming through concrete walls. (Block and poured concrete are porous wicks for water.) Check for in-ground water pressure against a subterranean wall, especially if the wall is at the bottom of a hill.

A musty smell is the first sign of mold!Check your bathroom and behind furniture and sofas positioned close to a wall. Clothes, especially leather, stored in poorly ventilated wardrobes, are often affected by mold.

If you don't eliminate the mold in your environment, you are in for a vicious cycle, which will ultimately lead to a chronic illness.

☯ DENTAL INFECTIONS

As described above, there are a lot of reasons for your immune system to be overwhelmed.

One of the most toxic areas in your body is your mouth. Not only is everything that enters your mouth immediately absorbed into the system, but it is also where many of us have serious problems.

It all starts with poor hygiene, which allows bacteria to grow. This warm and moist environment is the perfect breeding ground for bacteria and fungi, which stress your immune system dramatically.

Then there are tooth decay and matters pertaining to the bone and gums. Serious inflammations, bleeding gums, bone loss, ulcers, and cysts are very common.

Another problem can come from cavitations—holes in your jawbone that result from the extraction of an infected tooth. When the cavity is not properly cleaned out and the bone closes over the infected area, an internal inflammation accompanied by bacteria will cause toxic gases to be released into your body.

Then there are root canals, which are similar to an internal infection of the dentin where anaerobic bacteria live. The process of inflammation and infection of the pulpal and then the periapical tissues (around the root tip) will lead to the generation of many toxic chemicals. These include volatile sulfur compounds, such as hydrogen sulfide (H_2S) and methyl mercaptan (CH_3SH) which seep out into your body where your immune system must take care of it.

Finally, there are dental toxins from fillings and treatments. If you have mercury fillings, you are constantly absorbing highly toxic neurotoxins into your body, which have an adverse effect on your immune system. If you have dental sealants, you are continually absorbing Bisphenol A into your system, and this also stresses your immune response. If you go to a normal dentist, you will be exposed to hundreds of dental toxins. SO DON'T GO!

☯ IMPLANT INFECTION

REJECTION is an immune response in which our body recognizes something as foreign and then mounts an attack to remove it. This is an immediate, natural reaction if you have a splinter. The body begins to form an inflammation to increase the blood flow in that area, and the immune system starts to fight against the intruder.

If you have implants (teeth, breast, hips, joints), your immune system is activated. That's why, in many cases, you receive immune-suppressing medication so that your body will not reject the intruder. In a healthy body this normally does not cause too much trouble, but in a sick and weakened body it can be devastating—especially if your immune system is already working overtime. The two main risks are inflammation and infection.

☯ CONSTIPATION

Another war that constantly rages within your body involves re-absorption of waste material. In the case of constipation and bloating, bacteria and toxic gases are reabsorbed into your body from your intestines. This challenges your immune system as these particles are floating in your blood and plasma.

As long as your immune system is in good working condition, it will be able to clean this mess up with relatively little effort. But if your immune system is limited and weak, it will attempt to take a short cut and simply sweep the waste into a pile with the intention of cleaning it up properly when it has more time and energy. This means your immune system leaves little rubbish piles throughout your body, creating the perfect breeding ground for cancer.

Diet

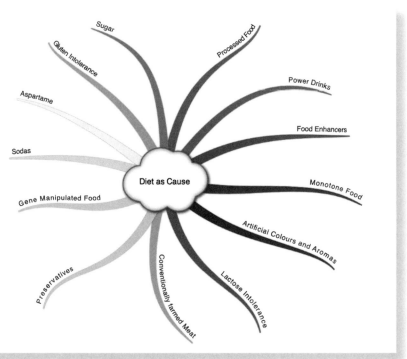

A proper diet provides energy, nutrition, strength, and power to your army of defense, but an improper diet causes your soldiers to be tired, malnourished, and weak. It demobilizes and starves your immune army and fills the body with junk that has little to no nutritional value. When you fill the system with many toxins, your immune army thinks they are under a toxic bombardment of the enemy which results in allergic reactions, a breakdown, and fatigue.

A bad, unhealthy diet always leads to inflammations, toxic overload, and deficiencies, as well as neurotoxic overload and stress.

☯ PROCESSED DEAD FOOD

You are probably familiar with the old saying, "You are what you eat." If you eat dead food, your body dies. If you eat junk, your body is junk.

It's that simple. Depending on your inherited stamina and strength, it might take awhile, but you can be certain that diet and lifestyle choices will eventually catch up to you.

Most of the so-called "civilized population" consumes more dead foods (cooked, baked, fried, boiled/broiled, sterilized, homogenized, microwaved) than raw or living foods, and the results are devastating. Statistics show a steady increase in all degenerative diseases. This illustrates that we are heading towards a massive health crisis where each generation will have an even shorter lifespan than the generation before them.

Dead foods must be preserved, which alters their molecular structure and energy. Therefore, they are NOT recognized as FOOD any more by your body but as toxins.

Considering generations of inherited genetic imprints, we are designed to eat food when it's fresh. It is meant to be eaten immediately, in its prime, living form to obtain the nutrients our body needs, such as minerals, trace elements, vitamins, protein, essential fatty acids, etc.

☯ SUGAR

A century ago Americans consumed 40 pounds of sugar a year. Last year THEY consumed 140 pounds. OUCH!

Here are 124 Ways Sugar Ruins Your Health:

- Sugar suppresses the immune system.
- Sugar upsets the mineral relationships in the body.
- Sugar causes hyperactivity, anxiety, difficulty concentrating, and crankiness in children.
- Sugar can produce a significant rise in triglycerides.
- Sugar contributes to the reduction in defense against bacterial infections and infectious diseases.
- Sugar causes a loss of tissue elasticity and function.
- Sugar reduces high-density lipoproteins.
- Sugar leads to chromium deficiency.

- Sugar leads to cancer of the breast, ovaries, prostate, and rectum.
- Sugar can increase fasting levels of glucose.
- Sugar causes copper deficiency.
- Sugar interferes with the absorption of calcium and magnesium.
- Sugar can weaken eyesight.
- Sugar raises the level of neurotransmitters: dopamine, serotonin, and norepinephrine.
- Sugar can cause hypoglycemia.
- Sugar can produce an acidic digestive tract.
- Sugar can cause a rapid rise of adrenaline levels in children.
- Sugar malabsorption is frequent in patients with functional bowel disease.
- Sugar can cause premature aging.
- Sugar can lead to alcoholism.
- Sugar can cause tooth decay.
- Sugar contributes to obesity.
- A high intake of sugar increases the risk of Crohn's disease and ulcerative colitis.
- Sugar can cause the changes frequently found in a person with gastric or duodenal ulcers.
- Sugar can cause arthritis.
- Sugar can cause asthma.
- Sugar greatly assists the uncontrolled growth of Candida Albicans (yeast infections).
- Sugar can cause gallstones.
- Sugar can cause heart disease.
- Sugar can cause appendicitis.
- Sugar can cause multiple sclerosis.
- Sugar can cause hemorrhoids.
- Sugar can cause varicose veins.

- Sugar can elevate glucose and insulin responses in oral contraceptive users.
- Sugar can lead to periodontal disease.
- Sugar can contribute to osteoporosis.
- Sugar contributes to saliva acidity.
- Sugar can cause a decrease in insulin sensitivity.
- Sugar can lower the amount of Vitamin E in the blood.
- Sugar can decrease growth hormone.
- Sugar can increase cholesterol.
- Sugar can increase the systolic blood pressure.
- Sugar can cause drowsiness and decreased activity in children.
- High sugar intake increases advanced glycation end products (AGEs) (sugar bound non-enzymatically to protein).
- Sugar can interfere with the absorption of protein.
- Sugar causes food allergies.
- Sugar contributes to diabetes.
- Sugar can cause toxemia during pregnancy.
- Sugar can contribute to eczema in children.
- Sugar can cause cardiovascular disease.
- Sugar can impair the structure of DNA.
- Sugar can change the structure of protein.
- Sugar can make our skin age by changing the structure of collagen.
- Sugar can cause cataracts.
- Sugar can cause emphysema.
- Sugar can cause arteriosclerosis.
- Sugar can promote an elevation of low-density lipoproteins (LDL).
- A high sugar intake can impair the physiological homeostasis of many systems in the body.
- Sugar lowers the enzymes' ability to function.
- Sugar intake is higher in people with Parkinson's disease.

- Sugar can permanently alter the way proteins act in the body.
- Sugar can cause liver cells to divide, and the liver becomes enlarged.
- Sugar can increase the amount of liver fat.
- Sugar can cause enlarged kidneys and produce pathological changes in them.
- Sugar can damage the pancreas.
- Sugar can increase the body's fluid retention.
- Sugar is enemy #1 of the bowel movement.
- Sugar can cause myopia (nearsightedness).
- Sugar compromises the lining of the capillaries.
- Sugar can make the tendons more brittle.
- Sugar can cause headaches, including migraines.
- Sugar plays a role in pancreatic cancer in women.
- Sugar can adversely affect a child's grades in school and cause learning disorders.
- Sugar can cause an increase in delta, alpha, and theta brain waves.
- Sugar can cause depression.
- Sugar increases the risk of gastric cancer.
- Sugar can cause dyspepsia (indigestion).
- Sugar can increase your risk of gout.
- Sugar can increase the levels of glucose in an oral glucose tolerance test over the ingestion of complex carbohydrates.
- Sugar can increase the insulin response in humans consuming high-sugar diets compared to low-sugar diets.
- A diet high in refined sugar reduces learning capacity.
- Sugar can cause two blood proteins, albumin and lipoproteins, to be less effective, which may reduce the body's ability to handle fat and cholesterol.
- Sugar can contribute to Alzheimer's disease.
- Sugar can cause platelet adhesiveness.

- Sugar can cause a hormonal imbalance; some hormones become underactive and others become overactive.
- Sugar can lead to the formation of kidney stones.
- Sugar can cause the hypothalamus to become highly sensitive to a large variety of stimuli.
- Sugar can lead to dizziness.
- Diets high in sugar can cause free radicals and oxidative stress.
- Subjects with peripheral vascular disease and high sucrose diets experience a significant increase in platelet adhesion.
- A high sugar diet can lead to biliary tract cancer.
- Sugar feeds cancer.
- The high sugar consumption of pregnant adolescents is associated with a twofold increased risk for delivering a small-for-gestational-age (SGA) infant.
- High sugar consumption can lead to a substantial decrease in gestation duration among adolescents.
- Sugar slows food's travel time through the gastrointestinal tract.
- Sugar increases the concentration of bile acids in stools and bacterial enzymes in the colon. This can modify bile to produce cancer-causing compounds and colon cancer.
- Sugar increases estradiol (the most potent form of naturally occurring estrogen) in men.
- Sugar combines and destroys the enzyme phosphatase, which makes the process of digestion more difficult.
- Sugar can be a risk factor for gallbladder cancer.
- Sugar is an addictive substance.
- Similar to alcohol, sugar can be intoxicating.
- Sugar can exacerbate PMS.
- Sugar, given to premature babies, can affect the amount of carbon dioxide they produce.
- A decrease in sugar intake can increase emotional stability.
- The body changes sugar into 2 to 5 times more fat in the bloodstream than it does starch.

- The rapid absorption of sugar promotes excessive food intake in obese subjects.
- Sugar can worsen the symptoms of children with attention deficit hyperactivity disorder (ADHD).
- Sugar adversely affects urinary electrolyte composition.
- Sugar can slow down the ability of the adrenal glands to function.
- Sugar has the potential to induce abnormal metabolic processes in a normal, healthy individual and to promote chronic degenerative diseases.
- IVs (intravenous feedings) of sugar water can cut off oxygen to the brain.
- High sucrose intake could be an important risk factor for lung cancer.
- Sugar increases the risk of polio.
- High sugar intake can cause epileptic seizures.
- Sugar causes high blood pressure in obese people.
- In Intensive Care Units: Limiting sugar saves lives.
- Sugar may induce cell death.
- Sugar may impair the physiological homeostasis of many systems in living organisms. In juvenile rehabilitation camps, when children were put on a low-sugar diet, there was a 44 percent drop in antisocial behavior.
- Sugar can cause gastric cancer.
- Sugar dehydrates newborns.
- Sugar can cause gum disease.
- Sugar increases the estradiol in young men.
- Sugar can cause low birth-weight babies.

Thanks to Creative Health Institute for this great list.

Sugar is the #1 killer today, and you can buy nothing in a supermarket, except in the veggie department, that isn't loaded with sugar. If you would just read the labels and know that 36 grams is equal to 144 sugar cubes, then you would understand what you are buying when you grab a bottle of BBQ sauce from the shelf. Plus it's the worst form of sugar possible—High Fructose Corn Syrup, from gene-manipulated corn, kills you slowly but surely.

☯ CONVENTIONAL FARMED MEAT

Conventional meat and poultry are usually fed with grains (such as GMO soy and corn). Carbohydrates fatten up livestock very fast and are, therefore, a lucrative form of producing meat.

Unfortunately, there are a few drawbacks in this business. First of all, the grains are laden with pesticides, herbicides, fungicides, and fertilizers which are then stored as toxins in the fat of the animals. Because of the high carbohydrate diet, the animal's immune system is very weak and needs a constant supply of antibiotics and other drugs to keep them alive.

These animals are also injected with synthetic growth promoting hormones, something you definitely don't want to ingest.

Australia has 700 accredited feedlots to raise grain fed cattle and 80 percent of the beef sold in an all major domestic supermarkets in Australia comes from feedlots.

In the not-so-distant future, the biggest problem we will face is antibiotic-resistant bacteria strains. Drug resistant infections have sky-rocketed over the past two decades, killing an estimated 70,000 Americans in 2009 alone. It's an emerging health crisis that scientists say is caused not only by the overuse of antibiotics in humans but in livestock as well. Antibiotics are being fed to healthy animals to promote growth and prevent disease.

We find antibiotics not only in the meat we eat but also in our waterways because of the runoff of crop fertilizers from farmland and manure.

The only meat that can be recommended is organic, grass fed, unpreserved meat that which comes from a reliable source. David Getoff refers to organic meat as "hormone and medication free and grass fed from birth to death."

☯ PRESERVATIVES

If you do not want to have bacteria growth, mold, and yeast in your food, you need to add preservatives and additives to preserve it. If you don't, your food goes bad.

Think about this for a minute!

What about the healthy bacteria in your gut? All those little critters which help you break down the food into all the nutrients that you need. What about the vitamins they produce for you? You are killing the "good guys" with these same preservatives that you use to keep your food fresh.

Salt and sugar are the most commonly used additives. Other food additives and preservatives are aluminum silicate, amino acid compounds, ammonium carbonates, sodium nitrate, propyl gallate, butylated hydrozyttoluene (BHT), butylated hydroxyanisole (BHA), monosodium glutamate, white sugar, potassium bromate, potassium sorbate, sodium benzoate, etc.

Here are a few, but certainly not all, dangers associated with these preservatives.

- Benzoates can trigger allergies such as skin rashes and asthma and are known to cause brain damage.

- Bromates destroy the nutrients in the foods. It can give rise to nausea and diarrhea.

- Butylates are responsible for high blood cholesterol levels, as well as impaired liver and kidney function.

- Caffeine is a colorant and flavoring that has diuretic and stimulant properties. It can cause nervousness, heart palpitations, and, occasionally, heart defects.

- Saccharin causes toxic reactions and allergic responses affecting the skin, gastrointestinal tract, and heart. It may also cause tumors and bladder cancer.

- Red Dye 40 is suspected to cause certain birth defects and possibly cancer.

- Mono and di-glycerides can cause birth defects, genetic changes, and cancer.
- Caramel is a famous flavoring and coloring agent that can cause vitamin B6 deficiencies. It can cause certain genetic defects and even cancer.
- Sodium chloride can lead to high blood pressure, kidney failure, stroke, and heart attack.

Traditionally, salt was added to prevent the growth of bacteria in MEAT. However, as meat processing methods improved, it was found that nitrates present in some salts gave meat its pinkish color while also adding a smoked flavor. For this reason, **sodium nitrates** are often used in curing meats to preserve them.

While a very small amount of nitrites can be tolerated in your body, excess amounts affect your health considerably. When nitrites are absorbed into your blood, they can react with iron to form methemoglobin. If this occurs, your red blood cells cannot transport oxygen anymore. This condition causes cyanosis, where your skin turns a blue-tinged color. In addition to cyanosis, headaches and dizziness are signs you may be experiencing this condition.

http://www.livestrong.com/article/477916-the-danger-of-nitrate-in-meat-preservatives/

☯ FOOD ENHANCERS

It's not a secret any more that ingestion of (or even contact with) monosodium glutamate and other ingredients that contain MSG are highly dangerous and cause severe health issues.

Brain damage, migraines, seizure headaches, cancer, heart irregularities, asthma, endocrine disorders (obesity and reproductive disorders), behavior disorders, adverse allergic reactions, neurodegenerative diseases, obesity, and retinal degeneration can all result from food enhancers.

Wow! That's what you give to your kids in almost everything you buy in the supermarket! Food enhancers are in everything.

Read the list of ingredients—not the label!

The following words will NOT protect you:

Fresh, All Natural, Traditional, Original, Plain, Pure, Gourmet, Finest, Wholesome Goodness, No Artificial Colors, Natural Flavors or Preservatives, No added MSG.

They use many different labels to hide the fact that they poison you.

Avoid 600 Series of flavor enhancers:

- 620 Glutamic acid
- 621 Monosodium glutamate, MSG, umami, E621 (in Europe)
- 622 Monopotassium glutamate
- 623 Calcium glutamate
- 624 Monammonium glutamate
- 625 Magnesium glutamate
- 627 Disodium guanylate, DSG or GMP
- 631 Disodium inosinate, DSI or IMP
- 635 Disodium 5'-ribonucleotides, I&G, nucleotides

Avoid MSG seasoning powders:

- Gourmet powder
- Chinese seasoning
- Ve-tsin powder
- Ajinomoto
- Accent
- Zest
- Chicken or other seasoned salt with flavor enhancers

Avoid hidden sources of MSG:

- Ingredients such as hydrolysed vegetable protein, soy sauce, or yeast extracts contain free glutamates that are essentially the same as MSG.

Free glutamate can be listed as:

- HVP (hydrolysed vegetable protein)
- HPP (hydrolysed plant protein)

And any combinations of:

- hydrolized, autolyzed, formulated
- vegetable, wheat, gluten, soy, maize, plant protein
- yeast (except in baked products like bread), yeast flakes
- yeast extracts (Vegemite, Marmite, and similar foods such as Promite, Natex savory spread, Vegespread, and Vecon contain free glutamates)

Free glutamate can also be present in added flavors in savory foods

- flavor(s)
- natural flavor(s)

Other forms of free glutamate include:

- kombu extract
- broth
- vegetable powder, tomato powder, etc.
- soy sauce—even without any additives, this is naturally very high in glutamates
- other sauces and seasonings, e.g. BBQ sauce, Worcester sauce, Bragg's all purpose seasoning
- all stocks and stock cubes

http://www.fedupwithfoodadditives.info/factsheets/FactMSG.htm

☯ ASPARTAME

Aspartame accounts for over 75 percent of the adverse reactions to food additives reported to the FDA. Many of these reactions are very serious, including seizures and death.

Aspartame is, by far, the most dangerous and irresponsible substance added to foods on the market.

Aspartame is marketed under several different names: "Nutrasweet," "Equal," "Spoonful," and "AminoSweet" and is also found in the ingredient list under Sweetener 951.

Aspartame is used in over 5,000 food products, prescriptions, and many beverages.

When the temperature of Aspartame exceeds 86 degrees F (30 C), the wood alcohol in ASPARTAME converts to formaldehyde and then to formic acid, which in turn causes metabolic acidosis. (Formic acid is the poison found in the sting of fire ants.)

Formaldehyde is grouped in the same class as cyanide and arsenic, both of which are deadly poisons.

It just takes Aspartame longer to quietly kill, but it is killing people and causing all kinds of neurological problems.

How often are diet soda cans kept in a hot car or stored in hot containers before unloaded into a warehouse? There are 90 different documented symptoms listed in the report as being caused by aspartame.

- headaches/migraines
- dizziness
- seizures
- nausea
- numbness
- muscle spasms
- weight gain
- rashes
- depression
- fatigue
- irritability

- tachycardia
- insomnia
- vision problems
- hearing loss
- heart palpitations
- breathing difficulties
- anxiety attacks
- slurred speech
- loss of taste
- tinnitus
- vertigo
- memory loss
- joint painThink of all the diet sodas you and your kids consume. Think of all the chewing gums and 0 calories cereal packs, candy bars, and foods you eat.

Aspartame changes the brain's chemistry.

> *Dr. Russell Blaylock, neurosurgeon, said, "The ingredients stimulate the neurons of the brain to death, causing brain damage of varying degrees."*

Dr. Blaylock has written a book entitled *Excitotoxins: The Taste That Kills.*If it says "SUGAR FREE" on the label—DO NOT EVEN THINK ABOUT IT!The best website to read about Aspartame and Aspartame Toxicity Reactions is:

http://www.holisticmed.com/aspartame/

☯   ASPARTAME MIXED WITH GLUTAMATE (FOOD ENHANCER)

Aspartate and glutamate mixed into one food or drink act as neurotransmitters in the brain by facilitating the transmission of information from neuron to neuron. Too much aspartate or glutamate in the brain kills certain neurons by allowing the influx of too much calcium into the cells. This influx triggers excessive amounts of free radicals, which kill the cells. The neural cell damage that can be caused by excessive aspartate and glutamate is why they are referred to as "excite-toxins." They "excite" or stimulate the neural cells to death.

It's the equivalent of running 240 volts over a phone cable—the cable melts and is permanently destroyed. That's what your kids do when they drink diet sodas. It hypes them up, pumps them full of sugars, and severely affects their brain's ability to function, sometimes referred to as "burned out." No wonder they are EXCITED while killing themselves.

This combo is super toxic for children.

The blood brain barrier (BBB), which normally protects the brain from excess glutamate and aspartate as well as toxins . . .

- is not fully developed during childhood,
- does not fully protect all areas of the brain,
- is damaged by numerous chronic and acute conditions, and
- allows excess glutamate and aspartame into the brain, even when intact.

The combo of glutamate and aspartame slowly begin to destroy neurons. The large majority (75 percent or more) of neural cells in a particular area of the brain are killed before any clinical symptoms of a chronic illness are noticed. A few of the many chronic illnesses that have been contributed to long-term exposure to excitatory amino acid damage include:

- Multiple sclerosis (MS)
- ALS
- Memory loss
- Hormonal problems
- Hearing loss
- Epilepsy
- Alzheimer's disease
- Parkinson's disease
- Hypoglycemia
- AIDS
- Dementia
- Brain lesions
- Neuroendocrine disorders

http://aspartame.mercola.com/

❀ ARTIFICIAL COLORS AND AROMAS

Food dyes are one of the most widely used and dangerous additives. While the European Union has recently placed regulations on labeling food dyes to inform consumers of the health risks, the United States and Australia currently have no such requirement.

Here are some of the most common food dyes used today:

Blue #1 (Brilliant Blue)

An unpublished study suggested the possibility that Blue 1 was the cause of kidney tumors in mice. It's found in baked goods, beverages, dessert powders, candies, cereal, drugs, and other products.

Blue #2 (Indigo Carmine)

Blue 2 statistically causes a significant incidence of tumors—particularly brain gliomas—in male rats. It is found in colored beverages, candies, pet food, and many other foods and drugs.

Citrus Red #2

This color additive is found to be toxic to rodents at modest levels and to have caused tumors of the urinary bladder and possibly other organs. It's found in the skins or rinds of Florida oranges.

Green #3 (Fast Green)

This dye causes significant increases in bladder and testes tumors in male rats. It's found in drugs, personal care products, candies, beverages, ice cream, sorbet, lipsticks, and other externally applied cosmetics.

Red #3 (Erythrosine)

Recognized in 1990 by the FDA as a thyroid carcinogen in animals, this dye is banned in cosmetics and externally applied drugs. However, it is also known to be used in sausages, oral medication, maraschino cherries, baked goods, and candies.

Red #40 (Allura Red)

This is the most widely used and consumed dye. It may be responsible for accelerating the appearance of immune-system tumors in mice. It also causes hypersensitivity (allergy-like) and triggers hyperactivity in children. It's commonly found in beverages, bakery goods, dessert powders, candies, cereals, foods, drugs, and cosmetics.

Yellow #5 (Tartrazine)

Yellow 5 sometimes causes severe hypersensitivity reactions and might trigger hyperactivity and other behavioral effects in children. It's found in pet foods, numerous bakery goods, beverages, dessert powders, candies, cereals, gelatin desserts, and many other foods, as well as pharmaceuticals and cosmetics.

Yellow #6 (Sunset Yellow)

This dye is believed to be the cause of adrenal tumors in animals and occasionally causes severe hypersensitivity reactions. It is also found in bakery goods, cereals, beverages, dessert powders, candies, gelatin deserts, sausage, cosmetics, and drugs.

http://articles.mercola.com/sites/articles/archive/2011/02/24/are-you-or-your-family-eating-toxic-food-dyes.aspx

☯ SODAS

Some people drink soda pop as if it were water—some even drink it instead of water. Sure, the primary ingredient is water, but with all the other "stuff" it contains, it has a toxic, poisonous, lethal, venomous, and seriously harmful effect on your entire body.

Soda pops (or carbonated soft drinks) contain an alarming amount of sugar, calories, and harmful additives that have absolutely no nutritional value. Studies have linked soda to osteoporosis, obesity, tooth decay, cancer, and heart disease.

We encourage illness and disease little-by-little every day by NOT **preventing** the cause. We try to fool ourselves but our bodies' cells can't be fooled with respect to the things we put into our mouths.

Phosphoric Acid: This may interfere with the body's ability to use calcium, which leads to osteoporosis or softening of the teeth and bones. Phosphoric acid also neutralizes the hydrochloric acid in your stomach, which can interfere with digestion, making it difficult to utilize nutrients.

Sugar: Soft drink manufacturers are the largest single user of refined sugar in the United States. It is a proven fact that sugar increases insulin levels, which can lead to high blood pressure, high cholesterol, heart disease, diabetes, weight gain, premature aging, and many more negative side effects. Most sodas contain more than 100 percent of the RDA regulated amount of sugar.

Aspartame: This chemical is used as a sugar substitute in diet soda. There are over 92 different health related side effects associated with aspartame consumption, including brain tumors, birth defects, diabetes, emotional disorders, and epilepsy or seizures. Furthermore, when aspartame is stored for long periods of time or kept in warm areas, it changes to methanol, an alcohol that converts to formaldehyde and formic acid, which are proven carcinogens.

Caffeine: Caffeinated drinks can cause jitters, insomnia, high blood pressure, irregular heartbeat, elevated blood cholesterol levels, vitamin and mineral depletion, lumps in the breasts, birth defects, and perhaps some forms of cancer—not to mention the lining used in the can which contains BISPHENOL A and is described in another chapter.

http://www.naturalnews.com/004416.html

☯ TRANS FATS

Trans fats are created from vegetable oils when they are hardened into margarine and shortening. This process is known as hydrogenation. It makes fats less likely to spoil, so foods will stay fresh longer, have a longer shelf life, and also feel less greasy. Trans fats or Trans fatty acids are also found in fried foods like French fries, fried chicken, doughnuts, cookies, pastries, and crackers.

The dangers of Trans fats lie in the effect they have on LDL cholesterol levels. Trans fats increase LDL cholesterol levels while reducing the amount of beneficial HDL cholesterol in your body. This significantly increases your risk of a heart attack.

The name hydrogenation already implies that during this process hydrogen is added. Because hydrogen is an element of Trans fat, both are responsible for an acidic pH.

At least 300,000 premature deaths each year are currently thought to be caused by Trans fats. In addition, experts believe that reducing the amount of Trans fats in **margarines** alone would prevent 63,000 heart attacks annually.

Probably the greatest danger of Trans fats is one that is not often discussed—it is the effect of Trans fats in **distorting the cell membranes,** as well as cell structures. The reason this effect is so significant is that when the cells are affected, every part of the body is affected.

Trans fats not only cause the commonly discussed health related issues of heart disease, diabetes, obesity, and cancer; it also has wide implications for a long list of body systems and functions, including immunity and brain function.

For example, the effects Trans fats have on cell membranes cause them to interfere with insulin receptors that are responsible for controlling blood sugar levels, which leads to diabetes.

Likewise, the danger of distorting cells and causing them to be unable to function properly is a contributing factor to the development of cancer.

☯ GLUTEN/ LACTOSE ALLERGENIC FOOD

In a healthy digestive system, undigested or partially digested proteins will be eliminated as fecal matter. However, if one's digestive system becomes weakened due to poor food choices, food intolerances, alcohol consumption, eating processed foods and sugars, as well as from the normal day-to-day stress of life, the ability of the body to digest proteins can become difficult.

Damage to the surface of our gut, through the various factors listed above, leads to inflammation and deterioration of this one-cell lining. As previously mentioned, this is called "leaky gut."

First of all, we cannot digest food properly anymore, and secondly, undigested or partially digested food gets directly into our blood stream. Because 60 percent of our immune system is located in our gut, our body starts to react through an increased immune response by creating inflammation. The natural defense mechanism is for our immune system to detect this partially digested food as abnormal and attack it. The immune system reacts with antibodies (IgG) and sensitivities. This causes us to be sick and inflamed.

Without a doubt, chronic inflammation is an ongoing strain to our immune system and makes us chronically sick in the long run.

A delayed hypersensitivity reaction happens mainly with allergens like gluten and lactose.

Gluten and lactose are the two main foods that can cause an allergenic reaction to the body.

In this case, the only solution is to eliminate all allergens because without the elimination of these foods, healing is not possible. The inflammation will steadily weaken the immune system and lead to a chronic overload.

☯ GENE MANIPULATED FOOD

There are still many questions about the safety of consuming genetically engineered or modified foods. Exposing humans to large amounts of novel proteins that are not a part of the natural food chain could cause unpredictable problems. There is no time to adapt because when the body does not recognize something, it is designed to treat it as a toxin or an intruder, and it proceeds to attack and destroy it.

Another concern with genetically modified organisms is the risk for allergic reactions. Problems with allergic reactions are difficult to detect because symptoms can take a long time to develop.

Let's face it. Most people do not care that they are eating genetically-modified (GM) organisms every day. They have been trained to have blind faith in governmental agencies and believe they are well protected. Most people laugh at you when you tell them they buy insecticides, which are grown in the very plants they eat. Last week, when we mentioned this in a conversation, a gentleman at the table got really upset. He was certain that all research was only in our best interest and that no one would ever grow plants which are toxic for us and then sell them openly on the market.

I guess Monsanto and other biotechnology giants thank you for being so ignorant because behind your back, they've succeeded in replacing 86 percent of US corn with their patented, insecticide-producing "Franken corn."The industry name for this Franken corn is "Bt corn," and the insecticide is actually produced inside the plant, so it is impossible to wash it off. This is accomplished by inserting genes from the bacteria Bacillus Thuringiensis into the corn.

Can you believe that these giants claim that the insecticide produced within the corn poses no danger to human health because it gets broken down in the digestive system? If it kills insects and bugs in nature then you can be certain it kills the bacteria and health flora in your gut.

Eating sprayed vegetables was not good, but at least you could rinse and wash them carefully and avoid a small percentage of the toxins. Now, there is no escape from food that has the entire amount of insecticide genetically grown inside it.

☯ MONOTONE FOOD

It's not only the toxins and manipulations that can be harmful to your health. You can also cause nutritional deficiencies by starving yourself to death and depriving your body of vital nutrients by eating only a small variety of foods.

Did you know that most Americans eat only eight varieties of food all year round?

Think of a printer with three cartridges: a red one, a blue one, and a green one. As long as all of them are full, the printed copies look good. If one of them runs out, the printer still works, but the copies look weird, abnormal, and SICK. Your body works in very much the same way. Every cell divides into new cells, and the old ones die off. All of the "ink" tanks must be full to produce healthy new cells.

Home Environment

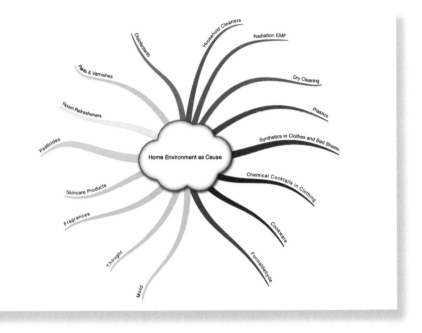

Household Cleaners

Radiation EMF

Disinfectants

Dry Cleaning

Paints & Varnishes

Plastics

Room Refresheners

Synthetics in Clothes and Bed Sheets

Pesticides

Home Environment as Cause

Chemical Cocktails in Clothing

Skincare Products

Cookware

Fragrances

Formaldehyde

Thought

Mold

☯ HOUSEHOLD CLEANERS

Hardly anyone looks at the amount of toxic substances we use daily in our environment. Women especially deal with them day in and out while cleaning the house, kitchen, toilets, and doing the laundry. Most of the household products that are sold in the supermarkets are loaded with chemicals that lead to serious health issues.

Ammonia, 2-butoxyethanol/ ethylene glycol butyl ether, methylene chloride, naphthalene, silica, toluene, trisodium nitrilotriacetate, xylene, bleach, and phsphates are substances found in many household products and are known to be endocrine disrupters, carcinogens, and reproductive toxins.

These products not only harm our health but are also flushed down the drain or sprayed into the air.

When we want to detox ourselves, we have to detox our environment and our home. All toxins add up, and, in the end, it is the sum of the toxic products we use that knock our bodily systems out of balance.

It is possible to buy plant-based, non-toxic cleaners or to make non-toxic cleaners yourself.

Use vinegar in place of bleach, baking soda to scrub your tiles, and hydrogen peroxide to remove stains.

Never forget every cell in the body has the ability to turn cancerous, and many do so on a daily basis. It is very important to keep this process in balance in order to have a well functioning immune system.

☯ FORMALDEHYDE IN FURNITURE, CARPETS, CURTAINS, AND CLOTHES

In 2011 the National Toxicology Program, an interagency program of the Department of Health, officially declared formaldehyde as a cancer-causing chemical.

Formaldehyde is a colorless, flammable, strong-smelling chemical that is used in building materials and to manufacture many household products.

It is used in pressed-wood products, such as particleboard, plywood, and fiberboard; glues and adhesives; permanent press fabrics; paper product coatings; and certain insulation materials. In addition, it is also used in resins used for office furniture, couches, baby furniture, industrial glues, foam insulation, paints, and paint thinners.

Many household cleaners also include formaldehyde: floor polishes, scouring cleaners, disinfectants, liquid cleansers, laundry aids, air fresheners, and carpet cleaners.

Formaldehyde is in other household items: wall hangings, carpets or throw rugs, textiles, plastics, and upholstery.

Personal care products such as hair straightening products, hair rinses, and cosmetics such as nail polish and hair gel often contain formaldehyde.

Baby products including shampoos, creams, and bubble bath are frequently laced with formaldehyde. It has also been found in baby clothes and bedding.

Toothpaste and body washes are also potential sources of this carcinogenic ingredient.

Clothing that is designated wrinkle-free or preshrunk frequently contains formaldehyde.

Formaldehyde is also a key component in the familiar "new car" smell of recently purchased vehicles.

Car exhaust and cigarette smoke also contain formaldehyde.

So what can you do to avoid exposure to formaldehyde?

Try to avoid most of the items listed above. Always keep your house well ventilated. Wash your clothing before wearing it. Buy only personal care products and baby care items that are formaldehyde free and certified organic. Be especially diligent with nail polishes and hair-straightening products, as both of these items may contain dangerous levels of formaldehyde.

Remember, it is all about the accumulation of toxins.
http://www.cancer.gov/cancertopics/factsheet/Risk/formaldehyde

☯ DISINFECTANTS

Scientists have known for a long time that exposure to disinfectants and antiseptics can cause bacteria to become resistant to them. Now they are finding out that Germs Fight Back!

The little nastiest have turned the gun on us, creating a weapon of their own out of the very thing that was supposed to defend us. They have become not only resistant to all kinds of disinfectants but have become more lethal than ever before.

Our ability to deal with normal germs has evolved over thousands of years. It's an evolutionary process where a balance is found by means of adaptation. Changing the germs into super monsters has destroyed this balance. Because our body has not been trained at the same time but has rather been weakened, this balance is lost.

In addition to this dilemma of disinfectants destroying our immune system, we have also killed all the good bacteria that we need to break down the food into nutrients to nourish our bodies. Our immune system has not been trained and now GERMS FIGHT BACK.

☯ DRY-CLEANING

The biggest organ of your body is your skin. Everything that comes in contact with it is absorbed directly into the blood stream. When you dress in clothes that have been dry-cleaned, you bring highly toxic chemicals directly in contact with your skin.

These toxins are absorbed by your body and accumulate over time in your liver. As the organ most responsible for cleansing the blood of any toxins, a struggling liver is unable to process an excessive amount of dry-cleaning chemicals. Unfortunately, conventional dry cleaners use a toxin that is particularly harmful to the liver.

Dry-cleaners routinely use the toxic solvent PERC, or perchloroethylene, to clean clothing. PERC is the most popular solvent and is estimated to be used in 85 percent of dry cleaners worldwide. According to the US National Institute of Environmental Health Sciences, PERC exposure can lead to headaches, nausea, dizziness, and memory problems. PERC's toxic byproducts include:

- Vinyl chloride, a proven carcinogen
- Carbon tetrachloride, a known liver toxin
- Phosgene, a hazardous gas that evaporates and can be lethal in closed spaces

- Trichloroacetic acid (TCA), used as an herbicide in the 1950s and 1960s which is deadlyEvaporated into the air, PERC can harm the health of anyone handling or wearing dry-cleaned items, including workers in the dry-cleaning industry and people who live near dry cleaners—but especially those who wear these clothes which have been saturated with these toxins.

Because a small amount of this chemical remains in dry-cleaned clothing, it can contaminate consumers' homes. The International Agency for Research in Cancer classifies PERC as a "probable human carcinogen." Already known to cause cancer in animals, several studies indicate that PERC exposure in humans increases the risk of esophagus, lung, kidney, and liver cancers. Other health effects associated with exposure to PERC are memory impairment, liver and kidney damage, endocrine disruption, menstrual disorders, infertility, and miscarriages. Clearly a toxic chemical, PERC can easily make its way into your environment if any of your garments are dry-cleaned.

Let me repeat again that not one chemical alone is the culprit for cancer. If you are handling these toxins every day, they might be the cause, but in general many factors together are overloading your immune system. The more you remove from your life the better your chances to recover.

☯ COOKWARE

Nonstick Cookware

A synthetic chemical called perfluorooctanoic acid, known as either PFOA or C8, is used in the manufacture of Teflon and nonstick pans.

Once heated, the coating of nonstick pans breaks apart and releases toxic particles and gases.

DuPont, the manufacturer of Teflon pans, has released data which shows the temperatures required to release these gases. Their results show that:

Teflon begins to emit gases at around 464°F (240 C).

At 680°F (360 C), Teflon emits up to six toxic gases, including two carcinogens, two global pollutants, and MFA (a chemical deadly to humans at low doses).

A test published by the Environmental Working Group shows that a Teflon pan can easily be heated to above 720°F (380 C) in five minutes during the normal process of pre-heating. Teflon and nonstick coatings become more harmful the older and more scratched they become.

Dr. Mercola mentions that other unrelated studies have also found evidence of birth defects in babies from PFOA-exposed workers. In 1981, two out of seven women who worked at a nonstick coating plant gave birth to babies with birth defects. He also mentions that Teflon may cause infertility.

> *Kenneth Cook, Environmental Working Group: "It's found in everything from newborn babies to whales in the ocean. It's indestructible, and lasts forever."*

The federal government considers PFOA to be carcinogenic—causing liver, pancreatic, testicular, and mammary gland tumors in rats.

Aluminum Cookware

Aluminum is a "reactive" metal, meaning that it reacts with salty or acidic foods to release itself into your food. Dietary sources of aluminum include cookware, containers, foil, and utensils. You can also face exposure to aluminum when the nonstick surface chips off a coated aluminum pan.

Aluminum is a causal factor suspect in Alzheimer's disease.

Stainless Steel Cookware

Stainless steel cookware is definitely the best choice in regards to nonstick and aluminum cookware. Unfortunately, all stainless steel has alloys containing nickel, chromium, molybdenum, carbon, and various other metals, there is a risk of metal leaching into your food, and there are allergen issues with it as well.

The best non-toxic cookware are glass, ceramic, (Le Creuset, Dr. Mercola) and cast iron.

☯ PESTICIDES

To fend off insects that could invade our crops, the industry sprays huge amounts of pesticides on the plants. These pesticides are then sold to end consumers or fed to livestock, which are then sold for consumption as well.

The bugs are dead, but the chemicals are accumulating in the end consumers. We are ingesting chemicals that were designed to kill living organisms. These chemicals reach the colon and remain there, making the colon toxic, slowly poisoning the body. These toxins kill our healthy gut bacteria and slowly overload our system to the point where it can't cope with the load.

The World Health Organization created the Codex Alimentarius Commission (CAC). Its purpose was to create international guidelines for food safety. In the face of these guidelines, the Codex Commission approved seven of the most toxic chemical compounds known to man for use as pesticides. Furthermore, they don't seem to be concerned about the accumulative use of these chemicals in animal feed and byproducts.

The seven dangerous chemicals approved by the Codex Commission are often referred to as Persistent Organic Pollutants (POP). "Persistent" because they aren't expelled easily, if at all. They remain in your body and accumulate in your liver and other organs until they poison you.

The problem is that all these toxins are not contained but constantly spread farther and farther. From the crop they are washed into rivers and into the sea. Organochlorine, one commonly used POP, runs off from the land into bodies of water and may be responsible for contaminating the world's seafood supply. Organochlorine collects in the fatty tissue, so fish, a meat that we used to recommend for their essential fatty acids, are also becoming unsafe to eat in regular quantities.

Even though most of these toxins have penetrated the produce and are stored in every cell, it is still highly recommended that you wash all fresh fruit and vegetables prior to consumption. Peeling is not recommended as the skin is where most of the nutrients are found, and, by peeling our fruits and vegetables, you reduce the nutritional benefits of our produce.

That's why there is actually no alternative to buying organic or spray-free fruits and vegetables from a local market. Support those farmers who care for your health and your wellbeing. They protect you and the Earth from greater damage.

☯   BPA AND PHTHALATES

Plastic has been part of our lives for over 100 years, and we can't imagine being without it. In 2002, about 107 billion pounds of plastic were produced in North America alone. Unfortunately plastics are not safe as most of them contain BPA.

What is **BPA**?

BPA is a hormone-disrupting synthetic estrogen. BPA mimics estrogen in our bodies and causes an array of health issues. BPA is used to soften plastic and to line aluminum cans.

BPA does not stay in the plastic container, cans, or baby bottles but leaches out into the food that is held by them. Especially when heating or filling hot liquids into the containers, the amount of BPA is drastically increased.

The Environmental Working Group tested canned food bought across America and found BPA in more than half of them at levels they call "200 times the government's traditional safe level of exposure for industrial chemicals."

We are not only exposed through liquids we drink out of plastic bottles, food we keep in plastic containers, and food we eat out of cans but also by touching items which contain BPA (toys, shopping receipts) as well as through air and dust.

The health issues associated with BPA are prostate and breast cancer, early onset of puberty, obesity, hyperactivity, lowered sperm count, miscarriage, diabetes, structural damage to the brain, and an altered immune system.

It is probably not possible to completely avoid our exposure to BPA anymore, but we definitely can limit our exposure.

Buy your food only in glass bottles. Buy BPA-free bottles and fill them up with your filtered water from home. If you have to store food, try to use glass containers.

In general, buy fresh produce and cook it at home. This avoids all kinds of containers and cans and is the better way to health.

☯ WHAT ARE PHTHALATES?

Phthalates are compounds used to make plastic materials like PVC soft, more flexible, and moldable. They are not only found in all plastics, plastic containers, sandwich bags, soda, milk cartons, juice containers, Styrofoam cups, and toys, but also in perfumes, toothbrushes, hair shampoos, hair sprays, paints, printing inks, sporting goods, vinyl flooring, footwear, outdoor clothing, and inflatable products. The new car smell is partly the pungent odor of phthalates coming from the plastic dashboard when heated by the sun.

Phthalates are endocrine disruptors and young males are most vulnerable to this chemical. Their young bodies are still growing and developing; therefore, their hormonal and reproductive systems are strongly affected by this toxin. In pregnant women, phthalates pass through the placenta to be absorbed by the fetus.

Health effects related to phthalates are:

- abnormal male sexual development
- male infertility

- premature breast development
- cancer
- premature birthasthma
- miscarriage.

A 2000 EWG analysis of CDC data, called Beauty Secrets, found that dibutyl phthalate was present in the bodies of every single person tested for industrial pollutants.

Be aware that phthalates do not have to be listed on ingredient labels. There is no way you can be sure that the product is free of phthalates when buying cosmetics. Phthalates are often used in cosmetics and personal care products to carry fragrances. They can be simply labeled "fragrance" even though they make up 20 percent or more of the product.

There are too many endocrine disruptors found in our environment. They play havoc with our hormone system, which regulates all our bodily functions. Our body is a very sensitively balanced system—one parameter out of control causes the whole system to begin to wobble. We do not know enough about how everything plays together, but it is certain that we should try to keep our system in harmony to function properly.

Again, we cannot run away from them as they are already in our environment (air, water, food), but we can stay away from most of the plastics at home, use reusable cups and bottles, have wooden toys for our kids, and use only organic skin care products. There are already healthy substitutes for regular paint, flooring, nail polish, hairsprays.
Fragrances

It smells so fresh!

Does it really? I don't think so. When I walk down the aisle of washing powders in the supermarket, I actually get sick.

Fragrances are not harmless, natural scents that smell good, but highly toxic chemicals which are absorbed through your lungs and skin.

Almost everything today is scented, from candles to cleaning products to upholstery to air fresheners to perfumes. All of these can potentially trigger allergic reactions which suppress your immune system. Artificial fragrances are among the top five known allergens. They can cause asthma and trigger asthma attacks.

Besides being uncontrolled and usually undisclosed, these fragrances contain highly toxic chemicals which, in large quantities, would be banned as toxic waste.

But one of the absolute worst dangers for your health is probably perfumes, colognes, and body fresheners which are sprayed directly onto the skin, where they are absorbed into the bloodstream.

Have you ever gotten a headache because someone sitting next to you is doused in perfume? The smell alone can cause your body to react with a serious sensitivity—not to mention if you bring these toxins directly in contact with the largest organ of your body.

Some people are highly sensitive to these toxins and feel dizzy, nauseous, irritable, confused, or fatigued when fragrances are sprayed into the air, on bodies, or furniture.

If you are weakened and want to avoid further stress to your immune system, I strongly suggest you avoid any form of synthetic fragrances. All of them contain chemicals which have been linked to cancer and all other degenerative diseases. Even though the FDA actually has direct authority to regulate harmful ingredients in cosmetics and personal care products, they don't.

The fragrance industry is allowed to regulate itself through a trade association known as the International Fragrance Association (IFRA). This association is supposed to be responsible for conducting safety tests to determine that the ingredients used in their industry are safe for use.

This would be the same as handing over the key to prisoners and asking them to guard themselves.

As most scents are attached to a product line and protected as a trademark secret, it's virtually impossible for these organizations to check these thousands of fragrances and their accumulative effects on your health.

The most dangerous chemicals used in these fragrances are synthetic musk and endocrine disruptors called phthalates.

The effects of endocrine disruptors, particularly during pregnancy, breastfeeding, and childhood are devastating. Animal studies on certain phthalates have shown these chemicals may cause:

- Reproductive and developmental harm
- Organ damage
- Immune suppression
- Endocrine disruption
- Cancer

Both phthalates and synthetic polycyclic musk fragrances have been found in the breast milk of American mothers, which proves that these toxins are absorbed through the skin and lungs and stored in fatty tissues. This has raised increasing concerns about their safety.

These fragrances are not all listed on product labels because they appear in minute amounts, but you just need to smell it, and, if it smells good (synthetic), then it's toxic. It's common sense.

The most harmful chemicals detected in samples of breast milk were:

- Xylene
- Ketone
- HHCB
- HHCB-lactone (the oxidation product of HHCB)
- AHTN

Tonalide is another common synthetic fragrance, which the Environmental Working Group EWG lists as a suspected endocrine disruptor. There's also some emerging evidence that it's a persistent, bioaccumulative toxin.

☯ RADIATION, MICROWAVE, EMF, WIRELESS

With many new developments, there are at least two sides in opposition, and they will argue which one is right and which one is wrong. Usually the corporate world, which produces the items, argues that it's all safe. They pay for doctor reports, university studies, and research papers to have reviews that are written in their favor. Patients, on the other hand, have less money, and they tend to voice their concerns on the Internet.

Electric fields are generated by an electric potential and magnetic fields are created by a flow of electric current. Combinations of these elements are called electromagnetic fields or EMFs.

EMFs are emitted by everything that uses electricity, like home appliances, lighting, computers, wireless devices, phones, transformers, home wiring, power lines, to name a few.

Those of you who have developed sensitivity to EMFs know that it is as debilitating as an allergic reaction to nuts. Your whole nervous system is on overdrive, and the body reacts like it is under an immune attack.

A reaction to EMF is not necessarily an intense experience. You can have headaches, nausea, sensitivity in the eyes, and other symptoms that are hardly recognized. Nevertheless, these symptoms are a sign of an over-stimulus of your nervous system.

It's really very simple. You are energy, and all of your bodily functions are regulated, down-to-the-minute electrical currents in your body. EMFs interfere with these impulses and send false signals to and from the brain. In fact, your whole body is like an antenna receiving countless interfering signals, which is perceived as stress.

Imagine what it would be like if all the EMFs were audible. In a German laboratory they modulated the frequency of EMFs into audible sounds which could be heard by the human ear. The sound was similar to screeching bats and scratching fingernails on a chalk board— dissonant, horrific sounds in many layers overpowering the ear.

There's a heated debate as to what electromagnetic field (EMF) level is considered safe. Because the experts have not come to an agreement, you'll have to decide for yourself.

Many government and utility documents report the usual ambient level of 60-Hz magnetic field to be 0.5 mG. Thus, any reading higher than 0.5 mG is above the "usual" ambient exposure. Many experts and public officials, as well as the few governments that have made an effort to offer public protection, have adopted the 3 mG cutoff point. The EPA has proposed a safety standard of 1 mG and Sweden has set a maximum safety limit of 1 mG.

Dr. Robert Becker, MD, has been studying the effects of EMFs for 20 years. He recommends a 1 mG safety limit in his book, *Cross Currents.* When electricians try to solve a magnetic field problem, they do their best to drop the level to 1 mG or below.

Dr. Nancy Wertheimer, PhD, an epidemiologist who has also been studying EMFs for 20 years, has been looking at the epidemiological data in a different way—she is trying to associate EMF levels with health rather than disease. She supports levels even lower than 1 mG. Russian researchers claim that 1/1000ths of an mG should be the standard.

The "BioElectric Body" states that there are several stages of health between "optimum wellness," "degenerative disease," and "cancer." Thus, we should maintain our own living and sleeping quarters at 0.5mG and below.

☯ PAINTS AND VARNISHES

Have you just painted the walls in your house and are irritated by odors, fumes, vapors, and off-gassing? Are you wondering how long will you be able to smell the paint and what the dangers and health effects are?

Different paint products use different ingredients, so it is difficult to comment on the health effects of paint in general. However, health effects associated with the paint will be significantly diminished as the paint dries. The best thing that you can do is to create conditions inside your home that will encourage a more rapid drying of the paint and ventilate the house to allow the odors to escape.

The reason you can smell the paint when it is wet but not when it is dry is because of the ingredients that make paint liquid. Depending on the type of paint, these ingredients are usually water-, oil-, or solvent-based. The chemical process that occurs during the drying of paint is called evaporation. Evaporation occurs when the liquid portion of the product changes from a liquid to a gas. These ingredients become dispersed in the air as they evaporate from the painted surface.

Just because it vaporizes doesn't mean it disappears altogether, though. For example, water liquid and water vapor are both still water—they just have slightly different properties. During the process of evaporation, another process occurs, called dispersion. The best illustration of dispersion is when you take a bottle of cologne and open it in one corner of the room. Within a few seconds, you can smell that cologne clear across the room even if the bottle has not been moved. That is because the cologne has changed from a liquid state to gas and dispersed (mixed in) with the rest of the air in the room. As the air flows through the room, it carries the odor of the cologne with it. Once you put the cap back on cologne (therefore removing the source), you will notice that the odor dissipates completely within a few moments because it becomes less concentrated as it mixes with the air in the room. Therefore, you're breathing in and smelling less of the cologne. This is what happens as paint dries. Eventually, all of the liquid in the paint will evaporate and be dispersed, and there should be little or no odor remaining.

Additionally, paint factory workers, construction painters, and furniture finishers face an increased exposure to paint- and solvent-related health risks. Paint factory workers are exposed to dangerous chemicals found in the paint itself; construction painters inhale toxic dust and pyrolysis products; and furniture furnishers can breathe in significant amounts of formaldehyde. Workers in these high risk industries may also face exposure to titanium dioxide, chromium, iron compounds, and, in some cases, asbestos.

Health Risks

Lung cancer, liver or kidney problems, contact dermatitis, bronchitis, shortness of breath, continual chest pain, or expectorating blood are associated with exposure to toxic chemicals in many paints and solvents.

☯ SYNTHETICS – BED SHEETS AND CLOTHES

When you snuggle into your bed at night, you probably never think it could cause more harm than good. Not even health-conscious people think of the dangers that are hidden in synthetic sheets and fabrics. But they should.

Synthetic fabrics are saturated with chemicals and dyes that cannot be washed out, making them lethal weapons.

Toxins in Your Textiles

During the production and processing of most synthetic underwear, towels, dress shirts, bed linens, blouses, and bras, these fabrics are treated with chemicals which you do not want to have close to your body. These chemicals are absorbed or inhaled directly.

Teflon in Your Pants and Underpants

In 2004, a new clothing additive was recognized as a serious health danger. The EMF advised parents to discard the clothing of their children and to buy natural fibers instead, if possible.

The danger was coming from perfluorinated chemicals (PFCs), which include the nonstick additive Teflon. To prevent the sticking and wrinkling of clothes, these chemicals are increasingly added to clothing because it makes them last longer. Most clothing labeled "no-iron" contains PFCs.

PFCs are cancer-causing, according to the US Environmental Protection Agency (EPA), and, if they declare something outright dangerous, it's probably beyond anything you ever want to touch.

Despite the EPA's warning, these "no-iron" and "wrinkle-free" synthetics have become a popular part of many school uniforms. I think if parents knew that the school uniform would contribute to their children getting cancer later in life, they would search for alternatives.

A chemical overload To create soft and flowing fabrics is not as easy as it seems. No one likes these scratching old pullovers that mum spun from her good old wool. That's why, in the early stages of the production process, chemicals are added to smoothen the process and to create a better workflow.

For instance:

- Chemicals are used to make fibers suitable for spinning and weaving.
- A formaldehyde product is often applied to prevent shrinkage. This product is applied with heat, so it is permanently trapped in the fiber.
- Petrochemical dyes, which are very toxic to the environment and the end consumer, are used for color.
- PFCs are added to make clothing softer, wrinkle-free, fire-retardant, moth-repellant, and stain-resistant.
- Commonly used chemicals include volatile organic compounds (VOCs) and dioxin-producing bleach.
- Nylon and polyester are made from petrochemicals, whose production creates nitrous oxide, a greenhouse gas that's 310 times more potent than carbon dioxide.
- Rayon is made from wood pulp that has been treated with chemicals, including caustic soda and sulphuric acid.
- Dye fixatives used in fabrics often come from heavy metals.

- Acrylic fabrics are polycrylonitriles, which are known to be carcinogenic.
- Clothing and fabric that are treated with flame-retardant chemicals, such as children's pajamas, emit formaldehyde, which is also proven to cause cancer.

There is clear evidence that all the previously listed chemicals are directly related to our present health concerns like cancer. These chemicals in synthetic clothes and bed sheets have endocrine and hormone disrupting effects.

Synthetic Fibers to Avoid

It's best to stay away from the following fabrics:Acrylic

- Polyester
- Rayon
- Acetate
- Triacetate
- Nylon

Anything labeled static-resistant, wrinkle-resistant, permanent-press, no-iron, stain-proof, or moth-repellant should also be avoided.

Your skin absorbs all of the gases, toxins, and other harmful ingredients used in synthetic fabrics. The skin is our largest organ and is able to absorb many substances through its big surface area.

That's why modern medicine uses nicotine patches, hormone patches for birth control or menopause, and morphine patches for pain control.

This clearly shows that the industry knows that any poison is directly absorbed via the skin and that they are poisoning you.

☯   SKINCARE PRODUCTS

Words ending in "paraben" are estrogen mimickers and chemical preservatives found in almost all body care products. They cause allergies in the form of rashes and have been detected in human breast tumors.

The following is a list

- DMDM hydantoin (can release formaldehyde)
- Imidazolidinyl urea (can release formaldehyde)
- Methylchloroisothiazolinone
- Methylisothiazolinone
- Triclosan
- Triclocarban
- Triethanolamine (or "TEA") (causes allergic reactions, skin dryness, eye irritations)

Ingredients that start with PEG or have an –eth in the middle:

- sodium laureth sulfate
- polyethylene glycol
- oleth
- myreth
- ceteareth (contain 1,4-Dioxane which is considered a human carcinogen)
- FD&C (colors)
- D&C
- 2-Bromo-2-Nitropropane-1,3 Diol
- BHA
- Boric acid and sodium borate
- DMDM Hydantoin
- Oxybenzone
- Phthalates, always found in perfumes, hair sprays, nail polishes, and all synthetically scented products such as shampoos, deodorants, perfumes. Beware of scented candles!
- Aluminum
- Propylene glycol PG

If you can't pronounce the ingredient, the best rule to apply is not to buy the product. Body products should be eatable to be considered safe to use on our skin.

Unfortunately, there are no government regulations regarding body care products and cosmetics. Companies can call their product natural or organic and still use petrochemicals as ingredients. There may be no certified organic or natural ingredients whatsoever. To be on the safe side, the product should be certified as organic by an official body.

The website from the Environmental Working Group http://www.ewg. org/skindeep is a fantastic site with more than 65,000 products to search for. Searching for specific ingredients is also possible.

Cosmetics companies may use any ingredient or raw material, except for color additives and a few prohibited substances, without government review or approval (FDA 2005, FDA 2000).

More than 500 products sold in the United States contain ingredients banned in cosmetics in Japan, Canada, or the European Union (EWG 2007b).

Nearly 100 products contain ingredients considered unsafe by the International Fragrance Association (EWG 2007c).

A wide range of nanomaterials whose safety is in question are commonly used in personal care products (EWG 2006).

Of all personal care products, 22 percent may be contaminated with the cancer-causing impurity 1,4-dioxane, including many children's products (EWG 2007d, CDC 2009).

Of all sunscreens, 60 percent contain the potential hormone disruptor oxybenzone that readily penetrates the skin and contaminates the bodies of 97 percent of Americans (EWG 2010, Calafat et al 2008).

Of all tested lipstick brands, 61 percent contain residues of lead (CSC 2007).

Authors: Jason Rano, Legislative Analyst, and Jane Houlihan, Senior Vice President for Research   http://www.ewg.org/skindeep

The following is a comprehensive list of carcinogens, hormone disruptors, penetration enhancers, and common allergens from the website of Dr. Samuel S. Epstein http://preventcancer.com/consumers/.

Dr. Epstein is also the author of the book *Toxic Beauty,* which we highly recommended if you want to know more about our toxic cosmetics and personal care products.

> *Dr. Epstein warns: "We are playing Russian roulette with toxic laden cosmetics and personal care products that we apply to our skin and to the skin of our infants and children, everyday."*

Table 1: Frank Carcinogens

Acesulfame
Acrylamide
Aspartame (NutraSweet)
Auramine
Bisphenol-A (BPA)
Butadiene
Butyl benzyl phthalate
Butylated hydroxyanisole (BHA)
Chromium trioxide
Coal Tar Dyes
    D & C
        Green 5
        Orange 17
        Red 3, 4, 8, 9, 17, 19, 33
    FD & C
        Blue 2
        Green 3
        Red 4, 40
        Yellow 6
Cobalt Chloride
Cyclamates
Diaminophenol
Diethanolamine (DEA)

DEA cocamide condensate
DEA oleamide condensate
DEA sodium lauryl sulfate
Diethylhexyl phthalate (DEHP)
Dioctyl adipate
Disperse blue 1
Disperse yellow 3
Formaldehyde
Glutaral
Hydroquinone
Lead
Limonene
Metheneamine
Methylene chloride
Mineral oils
Nitrofurazone
Phenylenediamines
Pyrocatechol
Saccharin (Sweet 'N Low)
Silica (crystalline)
Talc (powder)
Titanium dioxide (powder)

Table 2: "Hidden" Carcinogens

CONTAMINANTS

Ingredient	Contaminated With
Acrylate and methacrylate polymers	Ethylhexyl acrylate
Amorphous silicate	Crystalline silica
Alcohol ethoxylates • Laureths • Oleths • Polyethylene glycol (PEG) • Polysorbates	Ethylene oxide, 1,4-dioxane
Butane	Butadiene
Coal tar dyes	Arsenic, lead
Glyoxal and polyoxymethylene urea	Formaldehyde
Lanolin	Organochlorine pesticides, PCBs, ceteareths
Petroleum	Polycyclic aromatic hydrocarbons
Phenol ethoxylates • Nonoxynols • Octoxynols	Ethylene oxide, 1,4-dioxane
Polyacrylamide and polyquaternium	Acrylamide

FORMALDEHYDE RELEASERS

Diazolidinyl urea
DMDM-hydantoin
Imidazolidinyl urea
Metheneamine
Polyoxymethylene
Quaterniums
Sodium hydroxymethylglycinate

NITROSAMINE PRECURSORS

Brononitrodioxane (nitrite donor)
Bronopol (nitrite donor)
Cocamidopropyl betaine
DEA and fatty acid condensates
DEA sodium lauryl sulfate
Diethanolamine (DEA)
Morpholine
Padimate-O
Quaterniums
Sarcosine
Triethanolamine (TEA)

Table 3: Hormone Disrupters

PRESERVATIVES

Parabens
- Benzylparaben
- Butylparaben
- Ethylparaben
- Methylparaben
- Propylparaben

Resorcinol
Triclocarban
Triclosan

DETERGENTS (SURFACTANTS)

Disodium ethylenediamine tetra-acetic acid (Disodium EDTA)
Ethylenediamine tetra-acetic acid (EDTA)
Phenol ethoxylates
- Nonoxynols
- Octoxynols

SOLVENTS (PLASTICIZERS)

Bisphenol-A (BPA)
Butylbenzene phthalate (BBP)
Dibutyl phthalate (DBP)
Diethyl phthalate (DEP)
Diethylhexyl phthalate, or dioctyl phthalate (DEHP)
Dimethyl phthalate (DMP)
Nonylphenol (NP)

LAVENDER & TEA TREE OIL

METALLOESTROGENS

SUNSCREENS

4-Methyl-benzylidine camphor (4-MBC)
Benzophenone-3 (BP3), or Oxybenzone
Butylmethoxydibenzoylmethane (BMDM), or Avobenzone (Parsol)
Homosalate (HMS)
Octyl-dimethyl-paba (OD-PABA)
Octyl-methoxycinnamate (OMC), or Octinoxate

Table 4: Penetration Enhancers

GENTLE DETERGENTS
Diethanolamine (DEA)
Monoethanolamine
Triethanolamine (TEA)

HARSH DETERGENTS
Bisabolol
Disodium ethylenediamine tetra-acetic acid (Disodium EDTA)
Ethylenediamine tetra-acetic acid (EDTA)
Glyceryl laurate
Sodium lauryl sarcosinate
Sodium lauryl sulfate

HYDROXY ACIDS
Alpha Acids
  Alpha-hydroxy acid
  Alpha-hydroxycaprylic acid
  Alpha-hydroxyethanoic acid
  Alpha-hydroxyoctanoic acid
  Glycolic acid
  Glycolic acid and ammonium glycolate
  Glycomer in cross-linked fatty acids and alpha nutrium
  Hydroxycaprylic acid
  L-alpha-hydroxy acid
  Lactic acid
  Mixed fruit acid
  Palmitic acid
  Poly-alpha-hydroxy acid
  Sugar cane extract
  Tri-alpha-hydroxy acid
  Triple fruit acid

Beta Acids
  Beta-hydroxybutanoic acid
  Salicylic acid
  Trethocanic acid
  Tropic acid

Alpha and Beta Acids
  Citric acid
  Malic acid

SUNSCREENS
Benzophenone-3 (Bp-3), or Oxybenzone
Octyl-methoxycinnamate

NANOPARTICLES

Table 5: Common Allergens

IN HAIR PRODUCTS	
Shampoos	Formaldehyde, fragrances, lanolin, solvents, surfactants
Hair dyes	p-Phenylenediamine (ppd), p-toluenediamine
Waving solutions	Ammonium thioglycolate, glyceryl thioglylcolate
IN NAIL PRODUCTS	
Artificial nails	Methyl methacrylate
Nail base coats	Phenol formaldehyde resin
Nail varnishes	Resins (aryl sulfonamide, formaldehyde, methyl methacrylate
Nail hardeners	Formaldehyde
IN COSMETICS	
Lipsticks	Castor oil, colophony, pigments (e.g., eosin, azo dyes, carmine), perfumes, preservatives, propyl gallate
Eyebrow pencils	Pigments
Eye shadows	Colophony, preservatives (e.g., parabens, triclosan), pigments
Mascaras	Colophony, preservatives (e.g., triclosan, parabens), pigments
IN OTHER PRODUCTS	
Deodorants	Fragrances (e.g., cinnamic salicylate, jasmine, methyl anisate, balsam of Peru)
Shaving products	Propylene glycol
Depilatories	Thioglycolate
Toners	Arnica, coumarin, lanolin, oak moss
Face creams	Benzyl alcohol, lanolin, cetyl alcohol, parabens, propylene glycol, stearic acid
Sunscreens	Benzophenone-3 (oxybenzone), benzyl salicylate, courmarin, para-aminobenzoic acid (PABA)
COLORANTS	
2,5-Toluene diamine	FD&C Red 2
3,4-Toluene diamine	FD&C Blue 2
Acid Blue 9	FD&C Yellow 6
Acid Orange 3	Henna
Acid Yellow 6	p-Phenylenediamine (ppd)
Acid Yellow 10	Red 22
Acid Yellow 17	Red 2G
Acid Yellow 23	Resorcinol
PRESERVATIVES	
Benzalkonium chloride	Imidazolidinyl
Butylated hydroxyanisole	Metheneamine
Diazolidinyl urea	Methyldibromoglutaronitrile
DMDM hydantoin	Parabens
Ethylenediamine	Quaternium-15
Ethyl methacrylate	Thimerosal
Formaldehyde	

Table 6: Allergens in Perfumes and Fragrances

Alpha isomethyl ionone	Farnesol*
Amyl cinnamal*	Fennel oil
Amylcinnamal alcohol*	Geraniol*
Anise alcohol*	Hexyl cinnamal*
Balsam of Peru*	Hydroxycitronellol*
Benzyl alcohol*	Isoeugenol*
Benzyl benzoate*	Isomethyl ionone*
Benzyl cinnamate*	Jasmine absolute
Benzyl salicylate*	Lanolin and lanolin alcohols
Butyl phenyl/methylpropional*	Lavender oil
Cetyl alcohol	Lemongrass oil
Cinnamal*	Limonene
Cinnamic aldehyde*	Linalool
Cinnamyl alcohol*	Methyl coumarin
Citral*	Methyl-2 octynoate*
Citronellol*	Narcissus absolute
Clove oil	Nitro musks
Coumarin*	Oakmoss*
Eugenol*	Phthalates
Evernia furfuracea (treemoss extract)*	Resorcinol
Evernia prunastri (oakmoss extract)*	Vanillin
	Ylang-ylang*

Warning labels required by the European Union

(From the 2009 Toxic Beauty (BenBella Books) by Dr. Samuel S. Epstein with Randall Fitzgerald.)

☯ TALCUM BABY POWDER

One proven carcinogenic ingredient is talcum powder.

Talcum powder is processed from a soft mineral compound of magnesium silicate and is called talcum powder or just talc.

Talcum powder is a primary ingredient in baby powders, medicated powders, perfumed powders, and designer, perfumed body powders. Talc is used in smaller quantities in deodorants, chalk, crayons, textiles, soap, insulating materials, paints, asphalt filler, paper, and in food processing.

A woman's frequent talc use on her genitals increases her risk of ovarian cancer by threefold as stated in a 1992 publication in *Obstetrics & Gynecology.*

The capstone of this research case against talc came in 2003 when the journal *Anticancer Research* published a meta-analysis, or large scale review, of 16 previously published studies involving 11,933 women; a 33 percent increased risk of ovarian cancer was confirmed.

Nearly 16,000 women in the United States die from ovarian cancer each year, which means it is the fourth most common fatal cancer in women. By some estimates, one out of five women regularly applies talc to her genitals. This usage occurs either through direct application, or as a result of using tampons, sanitary pads, and diaphragms that have been dusted with talc.

Do not buy or use products containing talc. It is especially important that women not apply talc to underwear or sanitary pads.

As an alternative, you could use powder made out of cornstarch.

Work Environment

By now, it should be obvious that certain products are very toxic and can cause cancer, as well as many other health problems, especially if you work directly with these products.

The following two samples are only meant to be indicators of the dangers you live in. There are hundreds more. At your workplace, you can be in constant danger.

If we would just make a list of all the toxins that are used in building materials, we could scare each builder out of his business.

This must not mean that we cannot work anymore, but we can be careful, eliminate what's possible, and continuously detox so that we don't accumulate large amounts of toxins in our bodies over time.

☯ ASBESTOS

Asbestos is certainly one of the best-known products for causing cancer in the building industry, but there are thousands of other toxins. If you work in this industry, you know that there are warning signs and labels on almost everything. We have already discussed paints, but there are many other flame-retardants, preservatives, pesticides, and toxins used on a daily basis. These products are absorbed through the lungs and skin and accumulate dangerous levels very quickly. Daily exposure as a builder or contractor can be deadly.

☯ HAIRDRESSER

Second generation hairdressers are proven to have a 75 percent higher risk of cancer than any other area of the work field. That is an indication of how toxic these cosmetics, shampoos, and beauty products are. This profession has a lethal exposure to these toxins through the skin and lungs.

The fact that these toxins are handed from mother to child and accumulate in the baby means that it's definitely a time bomb waiting to explode.

☯ PETROCHEMICALS

Let me repeat this again.

You not only ingest toxins through the food you eat, but you also absorb them through the lungs and skin. Therefore, repeated use of these toxins will cause an accumulation within the body and cause disease.

In the case of working with petrochemicals, this danger can be everywhere.

There are thousands of petrochemicals in ink, crayons, bubble gum, dishwashing liquids, deodorant, eyeglasses, contact lenses, records, tires, food, toothpaste, ammonia, heart valves, car mats, and the list goes on and on.The manufacture and incineration of plastics such as polyvinyl chloride (PVC, commonly used in consumer product packaging and medical devices) is a major source of dioxin. Dioxins are also formed as byproducts of chemical processes involving chlorine, such as the manufacture of pesticides and the bleaching of paper.

Two of the most serious health effects of dioxin exposure are cancer and endocrine disruption, which leads to cancer. The petrochemicals that are so pervasive in our environment have especially adverse effects on rapidly growing fetuses and infants. Laboratory animals exposed before birth to one form of dioxin displayed physical deformities, retarded growth, and changes in physiology. Adverse effects on learning and behavior were also evident.

☯ HEAVY METALS

Heavy metals are metallic elements which are toxic or poisonous in very low concentrations. Examples of heavy metals include lead, mercury, cadmium, arsenic, chromium, and thallium.

Heavy metals naturally occur in the Earth's crust and to some extent enter our body via air, food, and drinking water. Unfortunately, with the ever-increasing pollution of our planet, the concentration of these heavy metals in our food chain, air, and water are increasing at an alarming rate.

Heavy metals poison us by disrupting our cellular enzymes, which run on nutritional minerals such as magnesium, zinc, and selenium. Toxic metals kick out the nutrients and bind their receptor sites, causing diffuse symptoms by affecting nerves, hormones, digestion, and immune function.

Heavy metals are dangerous because they tend to bio-accumulate. Bioaccumulation is an increase in the concentration of a chemical within a biological organism over a period of time, compared to the chemical's concentration in the environment.

The United States emits 48 tons of mercury a year into our atmosphere through coal-burning power plants. China spews 600 tons of mercury into the air each year, accounting for a great part of the world's non-natural emissions.

Lead and mercury are very toxic to the brain, nervous system, kidneys, reproductive system, and immune system.

A large percentage of the world's marine life is loaded with high concentrations of mercury. The World Health Organization (WHO) warns pregnant women not to eat fish because of its high toxicity.

According to the observation made by the internationally recognized medical researcher Dr. Yoshiaki Omura, all cancer cells have mercury in them.

Lead dust is created through industrial waste and can be inhaled and also gets into the soil and water. China has been found to use lead-based paints in the manufacturing of toys. Lead-soldered joints in plumbing can contaminate drinking water. Therefore, cities with old water mains may be contaminating the drinking water with lead.

Other sources of lead include vehicle batteries, ceramic, pesticides, cigarettes, art supplies, bullets, fishing sinkers, radiation shields, some ceramic glazes, and sewage sludge. Cosmetics may also contain lead. A study published in 2007 found lead in all 33 brands of red lipstick tested, including an all-natural brand. Even dietary supplements have been found to include lead.

The Australian website, http://www.lead.org.au, is an excellent source for providing information on lead poisoning and sources of lead and even sells a lead test kit for your water, dust, paint, toys, jewelry, ceramics, etc.

WWF's Helen McDade said, "In effect, we are all living in a global chemical experiment of which we don't know the outcome. Environmental contaminants are suspected to cause cancer, birth defects, immune system defects, reduced IQ, behavioral abnormalities, decreased fertility, altered sex hormone balance, altered metabolism and specific organ dysfunction. Every day children are exposed to chemicals that have not been tested for safety."

Heavy metals, such as mercury, lead, cadmium, copper, and aluminum have an affinity for tissue that is high in fat. It is the organs like the brain, bone marrow, and nerves that bear the greatest burden. So, in any condition that involves the brain or mental illness, nerve degeneration, bone marrow disorders, and immune overload, one should look for heavy metal involvement. Heavy toxicity may also exaggerate existing inflammatory conditions.

Hormonal Imbalances

One of the most common reasons why certain organs and body functions don't work properly anymore is hormonal imbalances. The following are the most common causes of these imbalances. Without the removal of the cause, there is no chance you can get better.

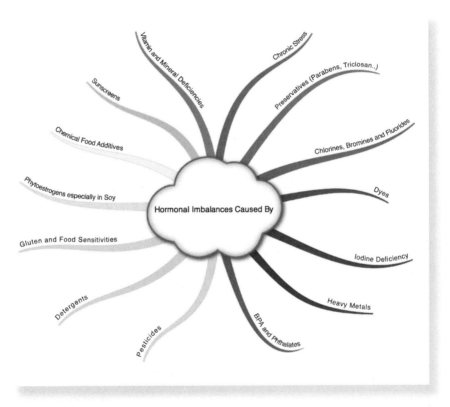

☯ THYROID

The thyroid is a small, butterfly-shaped endocrine organ at the base of the neck. The thyroid produces hormones that are used by every cell of your body to regulate metabolism and body weight by controlling the burning of fat for energy and heat. The hormones produced in the thyroid interact with all of your other hormones including insulin, cortisol, and sex hormones like estrogen, progesterone, and testosterone.

The fact that these hormones are all tied together and in constant communication explains why an unhappy thyroid is associated with so many widespread symptoms and diseases.

It is estimated that more than 20 million Americans have hypothyroidism, which is an under-function of the thyroid.

When the thyroid hormone is inadequate, the entire hormonal system is out of balance.

What are the factors that cause hypothyroidism?

- Chronic stress, which results in an increase of adrenalin and cortisol levels. Elevated cortisol has a negative impact on thyroid function. Thyroid hormone levels drop during stress.
- Environmental toxins such as petrochemicals, organ chlorines, pesticides, and chemical food additives affect thyroid function negatively.
- Bromines are especially common endocrine disruptors. Bromines are from the same halide group as iodine and fight for the same receptors in the thyroid gland. Iodine is a building block of the thyroid hormone. Unfortunately, it loses the battle and is replaced by bromine. Bromine is found in pesticides, plastics, bakery goods, soft drinks, and fire retardants.
- Iodine deficiency
- Gluten and food sensitivities can cause thyroid dysfunction because they cause inflammation.

Typical symptoms of low thyroid function are weight gain, lethargy, poor quality of hair and nails, dry skin, hair loss, fatigue, constipation, and cold feet and hands.

There are many more symptoms that can be associated with poor thyroid function as the thyroid plays a part in nearly every physiological process.

Your thyroid function can be tested with a simple blood test. The following panel of laboratory tests is what Dr. Mercola recommends:

- TSH—the high-sensitivity version. This is the BEST test. But beware—most all of the "normal" ranges are simply dead wrong. The ideal level for TSH is between 1 and 1.5 mIU/L (milli-international units per liter).

- Free T4 and Free T3. The normal level of free T4 is between 0.9 and 1.8 ng/dl (nanograms per deciliter). T3 should be between 240 and 450 pg/dl (picograms per deciliter).

- Thyroid antibodies, including thyroid peroxidase antibodies and anti-thyroglobulin antibodies. This measure helps determine if your body is attacking your thyroid and overreacting to its own tissues (autoimmune reactions). Physicians nearly always leave this test out.

- For more difficult cases, TRH can be measured (thyroid releasing hormone) using the TRH stimulation test. TRH helps identify hypothyroidism that's caused by inadequacy of the pituitary gland.

There are many ways to keep your thyroid healthy.

Suggested reading: *What Women MUST Know to Protect Their Daughters from Breast Cancer*, by Dr. Sherrill Sellman.

☯ ESTROGEN AND PROGESTERONE

Throughout life, women maintain a healthy body through appropriate ratios of estrogens, progesterone, and testosterone. A complex set of feedback loops determine how much or how little of each hormone is being made at any one time. This ongoing communication takes place between the brain, the ovaries, and the adrenal glands, acting in concert with all of the other systems in your body.

Fluctuations in estrogen can have dramatic effects on how we feel, think, and function. Compared to other hormones, estrogen is very tightly regulated by the body and is more powerful in smaller amounts than other steroid hormones. Estrogen has very important work to do in our bodies. It causes specific cells to divide and enlarge, controls reproductive cycles and pregnancy, prepares the breast for lactation, and influences the skin, the bones, the cardiovascular system, the immune system, and even the brain. Even tiny changes in estrogen levels can cause symptoms.

Hormones are continually changing from one minute to the next. Diet and lifestyle have a tremendous effect upon the entire neuroendocrine (brain-hormone) system—and directly impact estrogen and overall hormonal balance.

Excess estrogen wreaks havoc in your body. It can cause breast, uterine, and ovarian cancer.

Common symptoms of hormonal imbalance

- Irritability and mood swings
- Worsening PMS
- Headaches
- Sleep problems
- Irregular periods
- Heavy bleeding
- Problems with uterine fibroids
- Hot flashes and night sweats
- Breast tenderness, cysts, or nipple discharge
- Decreased libido
- Joint pain or stiffness
- Vaginal dryness
- Dry eyes
- Skin changes
- Heart palpitations
- Urinary incontinence

As women enter the perimenopause phase, the adrenal-reproductive hormone connection becomes even more pronounced. The adrenals are responsible for so much more than just pumping out stress hormones. One of their secondary jobs is to make and release sex hormones, to pick up the slack as production in your ovaries tapers off. If you've spent the bulk of your adrenal resources on chronic stress, by the time you reach perimenopause, there's little reserve for keeping peace in the sex-hormone camp.

Here's a simplified scenario of what happens when a woman who has been stressed out for many years transitions into menopause:

- The brain perceives stress.
- The stress hormones adrenaline and cortisol are released by the adrenals to help the body respond to the stressful event— whether it's emotional or physical.
- This occurs daily over many years, and cortisol remains continually high, resulting in symptoms of adrenal imbalance (see list above).
- During perimenopause, the ovaries naturally slow down production of sex hormones.
- Under stressful circumstances, the adrenals moderate stress first, leaving very few resources for maintaining sex hormonal balance.
- Menopausal and adrenal symptoms are intensified.

Stress is not the only factor of hormonal imbalances. Dangerous exposure to synthetic hormones in meat, birth control pills, hormone replacement therapy, and estrogen mimicking chemicals (phthalates, BPA, parabens) released in our environment are also contributing factors.

Reference:

http://www.womentowomwn.com

Dr. Sherill Sellman's book: *What Women MUST Know to Protect Their Daughters from Breast Cancer*A saliva test is the best method of monitoring your steroid hormones: progesterone, estradiol, testosterone, cortisol, DHEA and melatonin. Most doctors will still prescribe the blood serum test but the World Health Organization considers the saliva test to be the preferred method for accurately measuring hormone levels.

❂   ADRENAL GLANDS

The adrenal glands are tiny, walnut-size organs sitting on top of your kidneys. Adrenal glands manufacture and secrete steroid hormones such as cortisol, estrogen, and testosterone, which are essential for life.

The main purpose of your adrenal glands is to enable your body to deal with stress. They determine the energy of your body's response to every change in your internal and external environment. Whether they signal attack, retreat, or surrender, every cell responds accordingly. Your adrenal glands are the only way your body is able to mobilize its resources to escape or fight the dangers of stress and, therefore, survive. It is their job to keep your body's reactions to stress in balance so that they are protective and not harmful.

For example, the protective activity of anti-inflammatory and antioxidant adrenal hormones, like cortisol, help minimize negative and allergic reactions (such as swelling and inflammation) to alcohol, drugs, foods, environmental allergens, cancer, infection, and autoimmune disorders. These hormones closely modulate the utilization of carbohydrates and fats, the conversion of fats and proteins into energy, the distribution of stored fat (especially around your waist and at the sides of your face), normal blood sugar regulation, and proper cardiovascular and gastrointestinal function. After mid-life (menopause in women), the adrenal glands gradually become the major source of the sex hormones circulating throughout the body in both men and women. These hormones themselves have a whole host of physical, emotional, and psychological effects—from the level of your sex drive to the tendency to gain weight. Every athlete knows that steroids (adrenal hormones) affect muscular strength and stamina.

Even your propensity to develop certain kinds of diseases and your ability to respond to chronic illness are influenced significantly by the adrenal glands.

The more chronic the illness, the more critical the adrenal response becomes. You cannot live without your adrenal hormones, and, as you can see from this brief overview, how well you live depends a great deal on how well your adrenal glands function.

Stress can be triggered by many circumstances. A difficult relationship, money problems, financial hardships, air pollution, poor diet, lack of sleep, chronic disease, EMFs and inflammation are only a few of the possible causes.

As previously mentioned, the best method to monitor your steroid hormones is the saliva test.

☯ PANCREAS

The pancreas is located in the abdomen behind the stomach and is about 25 centimeters in length. The pancreas is a gland that secretes both digestive enzymes and important hormones.

The pancreas performs two important functions within the body.

Exocrine pancreas

The first function belongs to the exocrine pancreas. The pancreas produces digestive juices and enzymes to help digest carbohydrates, fats, and proteins.

Endocrine pancreas

The second function belongs to the endocrine pancreas. The pancreas produces the hormone insulin together with a variety of other hormones. Insulin helps to control the body's blood sugar (glucose) levels.

Insulin is secreted when your blood sugar is raised, and it causes the muscles and other bodily tissues to take up glucose from the blood to fuel their activity. Insulin also promotes the absorption of glucose into the liver, where it is stored as glycogen to be used when responding to stress or exercise. If the islets of Langerhans produce too little insulin, glucose levels in the blood rise which can result in diabetes as well as increasing the risk for a number of other problems throughout the body.

Unhealthy diets have a lot to do with pancreatic problems. Eating too many sugars such as candies, cookies, cakes, pastas, and even breads can cause an overload of sugar in the body. As the body breaks down these sugars, it does it so rapidly that it creates blood sugar imbalances that can lead to diseases like diabetes. This rapid rise and fall process of high to low blood sugar levels due to diabetes leads to the deterioration of the pancreas and eventually pancreatic exhaustion, which can be prevented by eating a proper diet.

There are many causes for the failure of our pancreatic metabolic function. Often more than one cause exists simultaneously within the cancer patient. Some of these causes are in the following list, and all must be considered as possible or ruled out as non-causative in each cancer patient:

- The pancreas fails to produce an adequate quantity of enzymes.

- We take into our bodies such large quantities of foods that require pancreatic enzymes for their digestion that there are no enzymes available for cancer digestion.

- Diet: incorrect type, amount, and timing of nutritional intakeThe nutritional components (vitamins, minerals, amino acids, etc.) are not available that are necessary for normal metabolism within the pancreas.

- We may fail to take into our diet enough minerals, which are essential to the release of the enzymes into activity.

- We may produce enough enzymes, but we fail to take into our diet enough coenzymes (vitamins) to make the enzymes work.

- The small intestine may fail to make adequate pancreatic activators.

- Obstruction of pancreatic secretion flowOften we produce enough enzymes, but the blood supply to a cancer area is so poor the enzymes we produce are not carried to the area.

- Proper pH balance (acid/alkaline balance) within the intestinal tract and/or within the cancer tumor massInfection: bacterial or viralChemical poisons within the patient's body from the environment, food chain, drugs, metabolic wastes, or medicationsManmade biologicals: Viruses or infectious agentsEmotional instability and/or traumaNon-absorption of pancreatic secretions (pancreatin) from the intestines into the body due to scarring or damage to the small intestine from various diseasesOur bodies produce anti-enzyme factors. The factors keep the enzymes from digesting our own bodies. Sometime we produce an over-abundant supply of these anti-enzyme factors.

- Balance: Instability and weakness of the autonomic nervo systemGenetic: Inheriting a very small, weak, or defective (ineffecti pancreasRadiation damage such as from therapeutic procedures, e
- Spiritual weakness

Symptoms of pancreatic problems

The symptoms of a diseased pancreas depend on the underlying cause may include:

- Pain in the upper abdomen
- Loss of appetite
- Yellowing of the skin and eyes (jaundice)
- Back pain
- Bloating
- Nausea
- Vomiting
- Digestive upsets
- Passing foul-smelling and fatty faeces

Endocrine disruptors

Endocrine disruptors are chemicals or manmade toxins which, when absorb have been shown to mimic the action of hormones. They can turn on, t off, or change normal signals. They can alter normal hormone levels, trig excessive action, or completely block a natural response. Any other bo function controlled by hormones can also be affected.

Hormone disrupting compounds are:

Pesticides, plastics, phthalates, pharmaceuticals, persistent organic polluta polychlorinated biphenyls (PCBs), dioxins, PVCs, detergents, and heavy me found in cleaners, dyes, cosmetics, personal care products, fabrics, build materials, mattresses, food, Teflon coating, disinfectant bleaches—the lis practically endless.

They are diffused throughout the atmosphere by the burning of industrial waste and leach into our groundwater from landfills and agricultural runoffs.

These compounds interfere with the essential inner workings of our cells. Measuring how dangerous they are has been difficult, not only because they interact in complex ways and at tiny concentrations, but also because literally every species has had some exposure.

Your endocrine system is one of the most sensitive communication networks—it influences all aspects of your health and well-being, including your reproductive potential, cognitive function, thyroid and metabolism, digestion, and hormonal balance. How an individual reacts to hormonally active chemicals varies, but one thing is certain: never before have there been so many diverse, manmade, and unregulated synthetics at work in our bodies.

Our body has an incredible detoxification system, designed to eliminate many toxic substances from our bodies. When we are exposed to very high levels of toxic materials, the body is simply overwhelmed.

Mental Causes

It is well known that any form of emotional feeling starts a chemical chain reaction in your body. Even fantasies and memories do that.

Think of an arousing situation and your body reacts.

Think of food and your body reacts with a gurgling tummy.

If you are afraid or sad, your body can even shake from head to toe. This can happen while you are watching a movie, where there is no real danger at all. Your body reacts to what you think, feel, and imagine.

As long as these emotions come and go, they are not bad at all. They help you to work through the situation. But when they become chronic and you can't resolve these emotions anymore, then they turn into a dangerous health risk.

Anything chronic is dangerous.

Severe traumas like the loss of a child or the pain of a separation or a shock from a robbery can get stuck in your mind and so become chronic. These situations have deeply rooted, emotional impacts, which, if not resolved, cause a constant suppression of the immune system and are perceived by the body as a permanent toxic influence.

Relationships

Relationships are probably the most intense battlefields of our emotional journey through life. They are active at work, at home, with friends, and even when you are by yourself. Yes, even when you are alone, you have to deal with yourself and all of your fears, desires, and fantasies.

These relationship problems are expressed in many different forms.

☯ RESENTMENT

RESENTMENT is one of the most debilitating emotional feelings. It's an ongoing feeling of anger, frustration, and pain, where, in your opinion, someone has done something wrong, or he or she has not fulfilled your expectations.

Emotions are rarely the only cause for disease as there are many contributing factors, but they are often the trigger for the system to collapse.

Suppressed or outspoken anger, fury, resentment, frustration, impatience, stress, excess, impulsiveness, and so on, often show in inner and outer bleeding, surgery, infections, high fever, absorption of high toxin levels, acute febrile, and infectious diseases.

In general, these emotions cause fever, inflammations, burning sensations, and hypertension. They are mostly responsible for liver and gall bladder disorders, including cancer.

Cancers of the blood, particularly leukemia, are knowingly related to suppressed anger. The most commonly recognized diseases related to these emotions are acne, boils, ulcerative sores, herpes, and venereal diseases.

Many people would argue that they do things out of love, but be not mistaken. Resentment always builds up if there is no balance. It's a drop each time until the container is overflowing. Resentment is stored in our subconscious mind and leads to chronic diseases.

☯ FEAR

Fear is always related to the fight or flight response and creates a great deal of tension. The natural reaction of the body is to prioritize. Because you need your legs for running and your arms for fighting, your body will shut down internal organs to increase blood flow to the extremities and muscles. It is a matter of survival, and all of the resources will be reserved to address the immediate threat.

This is an amazing feature available to our bodies on an occasional, short-term basis. A short burst of adrenaline can often provide the energy needed to escape danger, and that is why our bodies are designed to make these temporary adjustments. However, this is debilitating and outright dangerous in frequent or long-term conditions. Your body can't relax, and your nervous system is on overdrive until you completely exhaust your resources.

3 Main Fears:

- Fear of loss
- Fear of not managing
- Fear of not knowing

The diagnosis of cancer will activate all three fears. That's why emotional healing is mandatory to eliminate the fear factor in your life.

The best solution is to overcome the fear by intense study of the scary subject or object until you are familiar with it and it's not scary any more. Only when you engage with your fear can you overcome it.

☯ STRESS

Before we look at stress, we must clarify which forms of stress we are talking about.

Motivating stress

The first form of stress is the one that applies pressure to get things done. It comes in the form of time limitations, workloads, and when we have too many things to do at the same time. This type of stress is often born out of passion, provides motivation, and comes in waves. It is a repeated cycle of working hard until you have a breakdown and require rest and recovery. These waves tend to be less extreme with age.

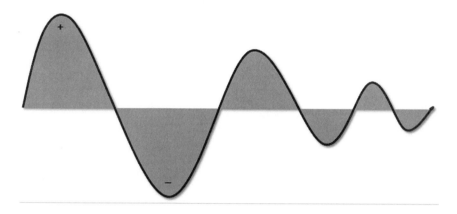

Debilitating Stress

Serious stress, which can cause physical problems, is caused if you have to surrender to:

- a duty you don't like to do

- a task which goes against your beliefs

- a husband or wife who is domineering

- a boss who bullies and harasses

- a belief or religion which you have to surrender to

- anything that prevents you from being TRUE to yourself

As soon as you **HAVE TO, MUST, SHOULD, HATE TO** surrender to the values, opinions, and beliefs of other people because you think you cannot speak up, change the situation, or stand your ground, you cause physical stress to your body.

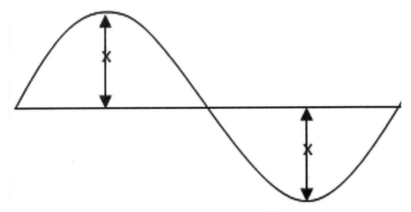

As mentioned above, that's not really bad if it's a temporary problem, but over time when you get stuck in your self-minimized situation, this can become the culprit for a breakdown of your immune system.

This is a very degrading situation that leads to all sorts of degenerative diseases.

☯ GRIEF

Grief is a normal feeling when you lose someone. You miss having them around, and the new situation "without them" needs to sink in. There are a lot of changes, and most of the time you need to find a new orientation in life. This part of grief wanes because life goes on, and there are many distracting factors.

But when grief does not subside—or even grows into unbearable pain—then something has gone wrong, and it's usually your memory.

From a vibrational point of view, grief is one of the lowest frequencies there is in the human spectrum of emotions. It's what many call rock bottom. And the health implications are huge.

Grief, depression, hopelessness, sorrow, and similar emotions are often related to old age, death, and decay. These emotions lead to chronic, wasting diseases and constitutional and congenial weakness. Under this domain are constipation, incontinence, low vitality, poor resistance, and poor absorption of nutrients. They cause numbness, stiffness, rigidity, and spasms. They also lead to arthritis, rheumatism, premature aging, osteoporosis, nervous disorders, paralysis, multiple sclerosis, Parkinson's disease, and cancer. Grief and hopelessness are closely related to deficiencies of vital fluids, dehydration, pain, and itch.

The intensity of your grief lies in your memories.

Most people remember only the good traits of the person that has passed away. My mother, for example, glorified my dad once he had passed away and only remembered all those things she missed. All of the negative traits, habits, and challenges were wiped out, dismissed, ignored, and erased.

Most people who do the same thing get stuck in grief fantasy, and this makes them sad. The bigger the fantasy, the greater the grief.

In a relationship there are hundreds of little things which are actually quite disturbing. Hair in the sink, dirty laundry left on the floor, lack of communication, grumpiness, different interests, cheating, domineering, lying, and worries are all part of a relationship, and there can be many more.

Even with kids there are worries, fears, anger, and frustration. They lie, steal, get in trouble at school, and disobey. When they are sick, there are hours of crying and complaining. They are seldom satisfied, and happiness is short-lived. When they have friends, they copy their behavior and follow the followers. In fact, if most parents knew upfront what they were getting themselves into, they might not choose parenthood as a venue for the next 25 years of their lives.

The problem with grief is that we are supposed to remember the good, and we have mastered this dogma with excellence, but it's a false memory that does not reflect the truth with respect to the person we have lost.

This is where emotional intelligence can save the day. When you identify both the benefits and the drawbacks of not having this person in your life anymore, you arrive at a neutral place in your mind. In fact, that's when you truly love someone because you don't accept only half of who they were, but you acknowledge him or her as a whole.

We will cover this subject in much more detail in our Emotional Healing Section.

☯ BULLY / VIOLENCE / ABUSE

People who are dis-empowered in several areas of life invite violence against themselves. Humans who are weak and helpless tend to attract behavior similar to the laws of nature where a weak member of the herd is cast out and rejected by the rest of the group.

Over the past few years, while working with many clients in this field, I realized that all of these clients who are dis-empowered in four or more areas of life have a bully at home or at work. Their low self-worth invites this kind of treatment.

Let's say you have no real purpose (**spiritual**) and no passion to motivate you to live. You have no money (**financial**) of your own and you resort to asking for help from your partner, parents, or friends. You have no education (**mental**) and no interest in obtaining knowledge and growing mentally. You are out of shape (**physical**) and do not care about your appearance, and you suffer from a variety of health conditions. You have very few friends (**social**), and none of them admire you because you have no achievements. You don't like your job (**vocational**), or you don't even have one. You only look after your family (**relationships**) and try to please them because you expect something in return.

This is a prime example of someone who is guaranteed to have a bully as his or her partner, parent, or child. The bully is nature's way of motivating these individuals so that they don't get comfortable in their miserable lives.

The most important observation here is that when a person is empowered in at least three areas of life, the bully vanishes. If they start earning money, care for their physical health, and learn how to apply some newly acquired knowledge into their work, the bully will miraculously disappear.

We will cover Mental and Emotional issues in Chapter 4.

Spiritual Causes

A purpose is like fuel in your tank. It motivates you to greatness and to overcome any obstacle in your way. NO PURPOSE—NO FUEL.

☯ NO SPIRITUAL PURPOSE

The spiritual purpose has nothing to do with any form of religion, but rather it springs from your heart.

I once had a great teacher who always encouraged me to listen to my heart. He said if you have a tear of inspiration in your eyes, you experience a moment of truth. This can happen when you watch a movie, listen to the lyrics of a song, or when you observe a situation in real life.

When this happens, analyze the essence of what makes your heart sing—the greatness that inspires you. If you are observant, you will find this life spark in many situations in your life. And once you follow it, your life is moved into gear. It's as if you are finally moving towards that which you are here for—your purpose.

Most people have never ever been in touch with this life spark. They live day-by-day, chasing a short-lived sense of gratification and never live out what truly inspires them. This is exhausting and drains their energy.

Having no purpose or not knowing what your purpose could be is a huge handicap in the process of healing. There is often no other reason to live than the fear of dying, which is a negative motivation. This might work for a while, but it's certainly not a replacement for having a purpose of your own. And because fear always comes with negative side effects, it's not a long-term solution.

Therefore it's a very crucial point to listen inside and to find one's purpose.

☯ LACK OF A WORLDLY PURPOSE

Similar to the spiritual purpose, which is far more in tune with who you are, is the worldly purpose. It is the motivation that drives you. Many say that our worldly purpose is expressed as PASSION and that it really does not matter what you are passionate about, as long as you are.

When you get up in the morning and you are inspired to do what you are about to do, you draw energy from a universal source. It's like tapping into the matrix and flowing with creation. This form of passion is life-giving; without this type of passion, everything is a drag.

We often observe a person who goes into retirement and shortly thereafter they fall ill and die. It was their passion and purpose which kept them going.

This worldly passion can change quite easily as it is often inspired by a void. That's why many have several different professions in their life or find fulfillment in each of their chosen tasks.

☯ NEGLECT OR DENIAL OF A PURPOSE

Not everybody is able to make their work their passion. Most people have to work in dull and boring jobs, and, in order to survive, they have to fulfill their DUTY. This is not pleasant and it's very tiring, but it's not really all that unhealthy.

Over time it can become a heavy burden, but often people compensate this drag with passion for a hobby. They refill their energy tanks by following a passion after work or after fulfilling their duty.

Surrendering your spiritual purpose, on the other hand, is deadly.

Probably the greatest pain you can endure is to know why you are here, but you are not brave enough to stand to your truth. Or you surrender to someone else because you think they know better than you do.

Denial or surrender of your spiritual purpose to some higher authority is expressed in growing resentment, frustration, and, in the end, even hatred. You despise everything you have to do, think, and express. In this way you poison yourself with your thoughts and emotions.

And even though it appears as if your anger is directed towards them, in truth it's directed towards yourself because of your own inability to separate yourself and to stand up for your beliefs.

This situation can be observed in most fanatically religious families, where one or more family members (usually the kids) have a different opinion about spirituality but are not brave enough to say so. They start the process by thinking "that's not true," which slowly grows to a state of "I can't hear that nonsense anymore," and, in the end, they have to either go and find their own truth, or they get sick and develop the most miraculous diseases.

Another example is when a woman knows that her purpose is to raise a child, and her partner does not want that. Most of the time, these women hope the situation will change over time, and, when it doesn't, they either leave or become sick.

☯ BELIEFS

Beliefs are very powerful and can have devastating effects.

The worst of all beliefs is that the doctor knows everything—especially when he has given you a death sentence.

Belief is a powerful tool as it triggers reactions in your body that can be miraculous as well as devastating.

Two robbers were surprised while breaking into a warehouse. They escaped into a freezer room to hide and waited for everything to turn silent. Then they tried to get out of the room but found the door locked.

The next morning, both of the robbers were found frozen to death. All pathology showed that the cause of death was hypothermia even though the room was defrosting, and the temperature was 12 degrees and increasing.

The mind accepts a placebo as a powerful remedy and heals by taking a sugar pill. So why should you not die if you believe the doctors when they tell you that you will die?

☯ TRAUMAS

There is an easy measurement for traumas.

If you can look at a life event and see the same amount of benefit as you can see drawbacks, you are completely balanced. The event is not affecting your behavior or emotional state.

- If the ratio shifts to about 3 to 1, you are emotionally opinionated.
- If the ratio shifts to about 7 to 1, you are emotionally obsessed.
- If the ratio shifts to about 9 to 1, you are mentally disturbed.
- If you can't find any benefits you are traumatized.

Traumas are off the scale.

Traumas such as losing a child in an accident can be off the scale. The trauma of abuse or rape is often off the scale. Traumas of watching someone being killed can be off the scale. These are situations where you can't see any benefit in what happened.

The judgment of where a trauma starts is individually different because we all perceive situations differently.

If you grow up in an environment where animals get killed on a regular basis to sustain the family, seeing a chicken being decapitated might not traumatize you. But if you come from a home where the meat comes from the supermarket, the same incident can be a very traumatic event.

In the same way, every trauma is based on your beliefs regarding right and wrong. If you grew up in Africa as a child soldier, for example, you would have different beliefs about killing someone else than you have now. These kids are proud when they kill as they climb up in their ranks. They get more recognition. It's the right thing to do. All their peers tell them so.

When people witness a traumatic situation, they will respond with a variety of emotional reactions which are repeated day in day out. It's like a tape that plays in their heads all the time. Everything they see activates their memories, so the same tape plays for years.

The problem is that these emotions and the memory of the incident do not vanish over time. On the contrary, they grow into a monster. The expression "time heals all wounds" might apply to the physical realm but certainly not to all emotional issues. In most cases, the complete opposite is true. With every repetition of the memory, the painful emotion is relived and re-imprinted in the mind.

If it is not dissolved, the person is forever bound to a painful memory. This leads to serious chemical reactions in the body, which in turn make you sick.

For example, cortisol is repeatedly released into your body, which suppresses your immune system and allows your body to get out of balance.

Therefore it's mandatory that these traumas are dissolved.

☯ DOGMAS

A dogma is the established belief or doctrine held by a religion, a particular group, or an organization. It is **authoritative** and not to be disputed, doubted, or diverged from by practitioners or believers.

As described before, a particular religion either coincides with your spiritual purpose, or it doesn't. And if it doesn't, it's absolutely unhealthy to stick to it.

One well known issue comes from the spiritual doctrine that if you do not follow a particular rule, then you won't go to heaven. Anyone who does not do this or that will be banished for eternity to live in darkness or go to hell.

How cruel it is to imprint such a fear into a child's mind—especially because we all know, on a soul level, that these are manmade rules designed to maintain integrity within the dogma. All dogmas are manmade. There are none in nature.

Unfortunately, these dogmas are very powerful, and to remain powerful they need to enforce their beliefs through violence. The church exhibited this behavior by burning all those who challenged the dogma. And even if the authority of such statements is not as obvious now as it was back in time, it's still very powerful: you might see the flaw in the system and you hate it, but you are not brave or strong enough to stand up against it.

Some of the most debilitating emotions involve self-minimization and self-surrender to a higher authority because they are mixed with hatred, anger, frustration, and resentment. It's the brewing of ingredients together that makes this cocktail so lethal.

There are three commonly known treatment options for cancer patients—burn, cut, and poison as they are referred to quite often.

These three treatments are called the GOLD standard, and about 90 percent of all doctors use these methods even though they have never proven to be successful, nor do they extend the life of a patient significantly. Most of the time they only deteriorate the patient's body and spoil the remaining time these patients have.

In the following chapter you will see that we have listed many other treatments which have been proven to be extremely effective in the attempt to balance the body and to heal almost every chronic degenerative disease.

None of these following treatments will, on their own, heal or cure cancer. They are a piece of the puzzle, and, if combined in the right order, can perform miracles.

CHAPTER 2

Treatment Options

Mandatory Treatments

You will have to adapt these different treatments into a plan depending on your condition and the causes you determined were at work in your body from the first chapter.

A high toxic load should be detoxed in many different ways.

A major deficiency should be supplemented through diet and supplements. A doctor, via IV treatments, should treat a severe deficiency.

Most of the treatments can be built into your daily routines.

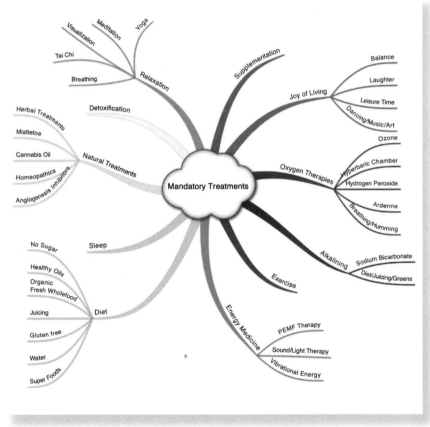

Natural Remedies

☯ HERBS

Herbs have been used for healing since prehistoric times.

Some important ones, which are traditionally used for anti-cancer treatments, are as follows:

- **Artemisia annua** (Chinese wormwood)
- **Viscum album** (European mistletoe)
- **Curcuma longa** (curcumin)
- **Scutellaria baicalensis** (Chinese skullcap)
- **Resveratrol and Proanthocyanidin** (grape seed extract)
- **Magnolia officinalis** (Chinese magnolia tree)
- **Camellia sinensis** (green tea)
- **Ginkgo biloba**
- **Quercetin**
- **Poria cocos**
- **Zingiber officinalis** (ginger)
- **Panax ginseng**
- **Rabdosia rubescens hora** (rabdosia)
- **Ashwagandha** (an Ayurvedic herb)
- **Bilberry**
- **Milk Thistle**
- **Chinese destagnation herbs**Herbs can also be used to aid in detoxification, the strengthening of certain organs, and stimulating the immune system.

Herbs stimulating the immune systems include the following:

- Echinacea
- Olive leaf extract

- Maritime pine bark
- Goldenseal astralagus
- Cat's claw and
- ElderberryHerbs with anti-inflammatory properties are boswellia and curcuma longa.

☯ MISTLETOE

Mistletoe is a widely studied alternative medicine for cancer. Mainly used in European countries, its extract is made from the European mistletoe, a semi-parasitic plant that grows on several types of trees.

Extracts of mistletoe have been proven to kill cancer cells in the laboratory, boost the immune system, and prevent the growth of new blood vessels needed for tumors to grow.

Mistletoe extracts are usually given by injection underneath the skin. The injection of the extract normally causes a slight reaction with inflammation, redness, and a slight fever, which is happily seen by the physician as a normal reaction of the immune system.

Mistletoe therapy is often called an immune provocative therapy because it makes the immune system react in a particular area; therefore, it stimulates the whole system.

☯ BLACK SALVE

Black salve, also known as Cansema or Amazon Black Topical Salve, is used to treat skin cancers and any kind of surface cancers.

The product is commonly classified as an escharotic, a topical paste which burns and destroys cancerous skin tissue very selectively and leaves behind a thick, black scar called an eschar (black, thick, dry scab).

There are many testimonials confirming that black salve eliminates the cancer, but, as with every single natural remedy, it's a tumor cell reduction and not a cure. Black salve does not remove the cause but rather eliminates the symptom.

Cansema is made out of powdered bloodroot and porkroot, zinc chloride, DMSO, charcoal, vitamin A, pine tar, and pascalite clay.

The FDA has taken an active role in banning products for use as a cancer cure, probably because it works so effectively and it's cheap.

☯ CANABIS OIL

For a long time, it has been known that cannabis oil contains cancer-fighting properties. Investigators are studying the anti-cancer capabilities of cannabis, as a growing body of preclinical and clinical data concludes that cannabinoids can reduce the spread of specific cancer cells via apoptosis (programmed cell death) and by the inhibition of angiogenesis (the formation of new blood vessels).

"Run From The Cure - The Rick Simpson Story" is a full-length video documentary that can be found on YouTube.

Rick Simpson stated:

> *"I have been providing people with instructions on how to make hemp oil medicines for about eight years. The results have been nothing short of amazing. Throughout man's history, hemp has always been known as the most medicinal plant in the world. Even with this knowledge, hemp has always been used as a political and religious football.*
>
> *The current restrictions against hemp were put in place and maintained, not because hemp is evil or harmful, but for big money to make more big money, while we suffer and die needlessly.*
>
> *Look at a proposal such as this: If we were allowed to grow hemp in our back yards and cure our own illnesses, what do you think the reaction of the pharmaceutical industry would be to such a plan?*
>
> *Many large pharmaceutical companies that still exist today sold hemp-based medicines in the 1800s and early 1900s. They knew then what I have recently found out. Hemp oil, if produced properly, is a cure-all that the pharmaceutical industry can't patent."*

In March of 2011, the National Cancer Institute quietly added a summary of marijuana's medicinal benefits to their treatment database.

Noted Statement:

"The potential benefits of medicinal Cannabis for people living with cancer include antiemetic effects, appetite stimulation, pain relief and improved sleep. Though no relevant surveys of practice patterns exist, it appears that physicians caring for cancer patients who prescribe medicinal Cannabis predominantly do so for symptom management."

Laboratory tests, conducted in 2008 by a team of scientists formed as a joint research effort among Spain, France, and Italy, were published in *The Journal of Clinical Investigation*. These test results illustrated that the active ingredient in marijuana, known as tetrahydrocannabinol or THC, can function as a cure for brain cancer by inducing human glioma cell death through stimulation of autophagy.

Marijuana is typically high in THC (delta-9 tetrahydrocannabinol)—the compound responsible for the plant's notorious psychoactive effect—and low in CBD (cannabidiol) content. Both THC and CBD are known as cannabinoids.

Cannabis oil ingestion is being recommended for the destruction of cancer cells within the body, not for recreational use. Healing results from ingestion of the oil from the marijuana buds, not from smoking the buds. The high heat from a burning marijuana cigarette can destroy the medicinal qualities contained within the cannabis buds. Furthermore, when smoking marijuana, carbon monoxide and tar are produced as byproducts of combustion and therefore increase the risk of introducing toxic elements into the body.

Please be aware that, in many countries, the use of marijuana is illegal. Merely having possession of marijuana can result in serious legal consequences.

☯ LAETRIL

Laetril, vitamin B17, and amygdalin are all three the same. Amygdalin is particularly prevalent in the seeds of bitter almond, apricot, blackthorn, cherry, nectarine, peach, and plum. The most common source of vitamin B17 is the apricot kernel.

Vitamin B17 is made up of 2 parts glucose, 1 part hydrogen cyanide, and 1 part benzaldehyde (painkiller).

When we introduce vitamin B17 into the body, it is broken down by the enzyme rhodanese. This enzyme is found in large quantities throughout the body, but it is not present wherever there are cancer cells. So rhodanese breaks down vitamin B17 into thiocynate and benzoic acid, which is beneficial in nourishing healthy cells. They form the metabolic pool for vitamin B12 production. The body will expel any excess via urination.

Because cancer cells do not contain any rhodanese, hydrogen cyanide cannot be broken down into harmless byproducts. When vitamin B17 comes into contact with the enzyme glucosidase, which is only prevalent in cancer cells, it causes a chemical reaction between the hydrogen cyanide and benzaldehyde to synergistically produce a poison that destroys and kills cancer cells.

Hydrogen cyanide has been proven to be chemically inert and non-toxic when consumed through food or a refined pharmaceutical, such as laetrile.

Dr. Contreras very successfully uses laetril in his clinic, Oasis of Hope, in Tijuana.

When buying apricot kernels, make sure that they are free of a mold called aflatoxin, which is very toxic and carcinogenic to humans.

☯ THE HOXSEY THERAPY

The Hoxsey therapy is an herbal treatment consisting of a topical salve, a topical powder, and an internal herbal tonic. This therapy was the first widely used, alternative, non-toxic cancer treatment in the present-day United States.

Harry Hoxsey, the founder of the therapy, opened his first official Hoxsey Cancer Clinic in Dallas in 1924. The clinic operated until the 1950s and became the biggest private cancer center in the world.

Harry Hoxsey was a renegade, self-taught healer who was very successful in treating cancer. Because he was treating patients but wasn't a doctor of medicine, he was constantly arrested. Harry Hoxsey is said to have been arrested more times than any other person in medical history!

If you want to know more watch the video:

"How Healing becomes a crime" available here:

http://video.google.com.au/videoplay?docid=5528328984547372206

Mildred Nelson, who was Harry Hoxsey's chief nurse at the clinic in Dallas, started Bio-Medical Clinic in Tijuana, Mexico. After her death, her sister carried on, and the clinic continues to operate and administer the Hoxsey therapy today.

In addition to the Hoxsey treatment, the clinic offers other supplementations for diet and nutrition, as well as chelation therapy.

The Hoxsey treatment is especially effective with skin cancer (including melanoma) and breast cancer.

Treatments at the Bio-Medical Clinic cost less than $4,000 for the therapy, no matter how long it takes. The clinic is only open for outpatients, which means accommodations must be arranged privately.

Bio-Medical Center
615 General Ferreira
Colonia Juarez

Tijuana, Mexico 22000

☯ CHAGA MUSHROOM

Chaga mushroom is a black parasitic fungus that grows on the living trunks of mature birch trees. The mushroom looks like burnt charcoal and draws its nutrients out from the living trees. After five to seven years, the Chaga mushroom causes the host's death; therefore, it is called "birch cancer" in Russia. The fungi digest food outside of their bodies by releasing enzymes into the surrounding environment, breaking down organic matter into a form the fungus can then absorb.

A look at the research on Chaga shows a similar pattern with respect to its effect on tumors.

Chaga has been researched as an antiviral, anti-tumor treatment for breast, uterine, and other cancers; diabetes; as a substance to increase immunity/longevity (strengthening the immune system and increasing the vital force); and as an immune amphoteric, for reducing blood pressure and slowing down heart rate.

Some experts claim the Chaga is the best anti-cancer mushroom of all.

Properties and ingredients of Chaga include:

- Polysaccharides that enhance the immune system, treat cancer, live, HIV, and other bacterial and viral infections.
- Betulinic acid to counteract viral infections and tumors. The anti-cancer properties of betulin or betulinic acid, a chemical obtained from birch bark, is now being studied for use as a chemotherapeutic agent.
- Triterpenes to lower cholesterol, improve circulation, detoxify the liver, and to treat hepatitis, bronchitis, asthma, and coughs.
- Germanium (a free-radical scavenger) to cleanse the blood, normalize blood pressure, and prevent tumors.
- Other nucleosides, phytonutrients, minerals, and amino acids including saponin, magnesium, chromium, iron, kalium, beta-glucan, inotodiol, isoprenoid, and others.

Chaga mushroom can be made into a tea or bought as a ready-made supplement.

☯ BLACK CUMIN

Black cumin seed oil from the Nigella sativa plant has also been found to kill cancer cells. The ingredient Thymoquinone (TQ) has anti-cancer properties that suppress the growth of and lead to the death of cancer cells.

Since 1959, there have been over 200 different studies at universities and laboratories regarding Nigella sativa. The Cancer Research Laboratory of Hilton Head Island, South Carolina, USA, conducted one of the largest experimental studies so far, proving that Nigella sativa oil had enormous success in tumor therapy without the negative side effects of common chemotherapy. Research found that it **increased the growth rate of bone marrow cells by a staggering 250 percent while inhibiting tumor growth by 50 percent.** It stimulated immune cells and raised the interferon production, which protects cells from the effects of cell-destroying viruses.

A study conducted in 1997, in Dhaka, Bangladesh, proved Black cumin seed oil to be more effective against many strains of bacteria than antibiotics.

Black cumin seed oil capsules were used in a study at I.I.M.E.R., Panama City, Florida, to reveal that the majority of people who took Black cumin seed oil displayed a 72 percent increase in helper-to-suppressor T-cell ratio, as well as an increase in natural killer cell functional activity.

Black cumin seed oil could play an important role in cancer treatment.

☯ CURCUMIN

Turmeric or Curcuma longa is a spice made out of a plant root. It is widely used as a food coloring and is one of the principal ingredients in curry powder.

The active ingredient in turmeric is curcumin, which has anti-inflammatory, antioxidant, and anti-tumor properties. Curcumin makes up 2 to 6 percent of the spice. There has been a substantial amount of research on turmeric's anti-cancer effectiveness, which proves that it has potential in the treatment of various forms of cancer, including prostate, breast, skin, and colon.

Turmeric has demonstrated an ability to inhibit tumor growth and stimulate apoptosis, an intracellular mechanism for cells of all types to "kill" themselves.

The active ingredient in turmeric can enhance the cancer-fighting power of treatment with TRAIL, a naturally occurring molecule that helps kill cancer cells. TRAIL stands for tumor necrosis factor-related apoptosis-inducing ligand. In an experiment with human prostate cancer cells in a laboratory dish, the combination treatment killed off two to three times more cells than either treatment alone.

Curcumin can suppress tumor blood vessel growth. This process, called anti-angiogenesis, can have a strangling effect on tumors. Researchers from the James P. Wilmot Cancer Center, through a study of mice, have discovered that curcumin may protect skin from the burns and blisters that often occur during radiation treatment.

Laboratory tests also revealed that curcumin made melanoma skin cancer cells more likely to self-destruct in a process known as apoptosis.

The best way to take curcumin is in its standardized 95 percent form. Curcumin is not easily absorbed into the blood stream; therefore, manufacturers add piperine to improve the absorption. Please be cautious when taking piperine in conjunction with other medications as it can also have a spiking effect on prescription drugs.

☯ GLUTATHIONE

Glutathione is an important intercellular antioxidant that plays a vital role in drug detoxification (liver detox) or elimination and in protecting against cellular damage by free radicals and toxins. It also plays a crucial role in diverse biological processes from protein synthesis to enzyme catalysis, growth and division, functioning of immune cells, and many more.

Glutathione selectively stimulates apoptosis (cell death) of malignant cells while leaving healthy cells unaffected.

Glutathione concentrations are sensitive to diet and nutritional status. As we age, our ability to produce glutathione drastically diminishes, which makes it hard to keep up with the demand posed by oxidative stress.

Glutathione cannot be raised significantly by oral consumption of L-Glutathione or Liposomal Glutathione, but it can be raised through glutathione injections. Unfortunately, these treatments are very expensive and last for only a few hours after the initial injection. The best way to raise glutathione naturally is through:

Spirulina is very effective in raising glutathione levels because it delivers all the essential and non-essential amino acids, which are needed for glutathione production.

Natural Whey Protein Powder contains three amino acids—cysteine, glycine, and glutamic—which are needed by the body to produce glutathione.

☯ MMS MIRACLE MINERAL SOLUTION

Miracle Mineral Supplement (Miracle Mineral Solution) is a well-known mineral solution and a water purifier that produces a compound approved as a water purifier in many municipal water systems. Activated Miracle Mineral Solution is harnessed by the immune system to safely obliterate pathogens in the human body.

MMS is sodium chlorite ($NaClO2$) 28 percent. Combining with acid briefly produces chlorous acid ($HClO2$), which in sequential steps oxidizes ambient chlorite ($ClO2-$) to create chlorine dioxide ($ClO2$).

As proven through research, chlorine dioxide is much safer than chlorine. It is selective for pathogens and does not create carcinogenic compounds, which chlorine does.

In 1999, the American Society of Analytical Chemists stated that chlorine dioxide is the most powerful pathogen killer known to man.

Miracle Mineral Supplement does not do the curing; it simply kills the pathogens that kill or diminish the power of the person's immune system. This enables the immune system to kick in and clear out the diseased cells so that the body can heal itself.

For this reason, it is also recommended (if desired) to take some sort of probiotic to help build your body's own immune system.

Jim Humble, the man who discovered MMS, suggests that our natural immune system cures our ailments. Only the body can heal the body. Humble has treated and cured over 75,000 malaria victims in Malawi, Africa. So far, MMS has a 100 percent cure rate for malaria.

The pathogen-fighting action of chlorine dioxide eventually results in Herxheimer reaction. This occurs when bacteria die and large amounts of toxins are released into the body because of the antibiotic treatment or fast detoxification.

This explains why most people get the impression that chlorine dioxide supplements tend to worsen their condition. This is an unpleasant feeling that usually consists of nausea and diarrhea caused by "die-off." Die-off refers to the pathogens in your body that are killed or destroyed by the CLO2 (chlorine dioxide—activated MMS). As these pathogens "die off," the symptoms can become more severe.

The more pathogens that are present, the stronger or earlier the Herxheimer reaction will be. In simple terms, the sicker you are (or the more you have wrong with you), the more intense your reaction may be.

The standard MMS protocol can be found here:

http://www.miraclemineral.org/important-info/

MMS kills pathogens but doesn't harm anything that is supposed to be there, such as intestinal flora. This is an important distinction as antibiotics are indiscriminate and kill what is supposed to be there along with what is not.

❦ HOMEOPATHICS

Homeopathy was started 200 years ago by a German physician named Samuel Hahnemann and is still practiced with great success worldwide.

The basic principles of homeopathic remedies are stimulating the body's own natural healing processes. Symptoms are not going to simply be suppressed as homeopathy considers the state of the whole individual—physical, mental, and emotional.

The system incorporates three important points, which are the law of "Like Cures Like," "Minimal Dose," and the "Single Remedy."For example, "Like Cures Like" means that the symptoms of your cold are similar to mercury poisoning which would mean that mercury would be the remedy. It has to be perfectly matched to your cold symptoms—where it occurs, what brings it on, what type of pain it is, what aggravates it, what makes it feel worse, your state of mind, and any other symptoms you are experiencing.

The remedy itself has many symptoms associated with it. The physical, mental, and emotional symptoms need to fit perfectly to the symptoms experienced by the patient. Herein lies the difficulty of choosing the right remedy, which takes time and expertise.

"Minimal Dose" means that the medicines, which can be found mostly in plants but also in minerals, animals, and toxins, are potentized by progressive dilutions; the higher the dilution, the stronger the remedy. After the homeopathic potency of 12C, there is no evident molecule of the original medicine found in the remedy. Nevertheless, in spite of the fact it has little or poor accepted scientific explanation behind it, it is used successfully to cure diseases including cancer.

The "Single Remedy" means that there is only one specific remedy that best fits all of your symptoms and is able to cure your illness. It can sometimes take a while to find this special single remedy, and some other remedies need to be taken first. It is literally like peeling off layers to get down to the original cause, clearly revealing the perfect remedy for the symptoms associated with the disease.

There are many beneficial factors in homeopathic remedies. When the correct remedy is taken, results can be rapid, complete, and permanent. Homeopathy is completely safe. Even babies and pregnant women can use homeopathic remedies without the dangerous risk of side effects. Homeopathic remedies can also be taken alongside other medications without producing unwanted side effects.

Homeopathic remedies will work in harmony with your immune system unlike other conventional medicines, which suppress the immune system. But the most important benefit is that homeopathic remedies are holistic; therefore, they address the cause and not the symptoms.

However, it is important that homeopathic remedies are prescribed by an experienced physician and not through self-diagnosis. The concept of homeopathy is too complex to be understood out of a book, weekend workshop, or an iPhone application.

☯ ANGIOGENISIS INHIBITORS

The biological process called angiogenesis is the process of building new blood vessels to supply the tumor with nutrition. We all constantly produce cancer cells in our body, and the danger of actually developing cancer occurs only when the cancer cells manage to get their own blood supply.

Anti-angiogenesis has just the opposite effect, where nutrients are preventing the formation of new blood vessels. Luckily, nature provides us with many foods and herbs that have anti-angiogenesis properties. These foods boost our immune system and prevent the tumor from dogging on.

Naturally Occurring Angiogenic Substances:

- Green tea
- Blackberries
- Raspberries
- Blueberries
- Apples

- Bok Choy
- Ginseng
- Maitake mushroom
- Licorice
- Turmeric
- Nutmeg
- Artichokes
- Parsley
- Garlic
- Tomato
- Olive oil
- Dark chocolate
- Kale
- Brussels sprouts
- Cauliflower

There are also many pharmaceutical anti-angiogenesis inhibitors, but they need to be prescribed by a doctor and carefully monitored. Most of them have severe side effects which need to be addressed.

Natural inhibitors do not have any adverse side effects and will not cause any harm to the patient. However, reasonable caution must be taken with the dosage amount—especially with garlic as it is known to have an adverse effect on your love life.

Diet

Diet is one of the most difficult problems we all have to face. There are so many recommendations out there promoting contradicting concepts that it's clear that many patients easily get confused.

Which diet is the best? The Atkins diet, a whole food diet, a vegetarian diet, a raw vegan diet, blood group diets, a metabolic diet . . .

The answer lies within the fact that we are all different, so the "One Diet Fits All" rule is not applicable.

However, there are certain important elements to incorporate into a cancer diet.

☯ FIRST OF ALL, SUGAR FEEDS CANCER.

Fifty years ago, the German researcher Dr. Otto Warburg discovered that cancer cells have a different energy metabolism compared to healthy cells. They use glucose and fructose as a fuel to produce energy. Cancer cells have around 70 insulin receptors compared to normal cells which have just four.

This means all sugars promote the growth of cancer, and fructose is the most dangerous one.

Research studies have found fructose guilty of inhibiting the action of white blood cells, which are one of the key elements of your immune system.

These studies have shown that eating or drinking 100 grams (8 tbsp) of processed sugar, the equivalent of a typical can of soda, can reduce the ability of your white blood cells to kill germs by 40 percent!

Sugar suppresses your immune system for several hours after consumption. The immune-suppressing effect of sugar starts fewer than 30 minutes after eating it and can last up to five hours.

Therefore, eliminating sugar from your diet is a mandatory action to heal yourself from any kind of cancer or disease.

When we talk about sugar, we are referring to every form of sugar. That includes white sugar, brown sugar, golden syrup, maple syrup, honey, agave syrup, and worst of all, HFCS (High Fructose Corn Syrup) that is used in almost all processed foods.

There many foods that are directly converted into sugar by your body. That's why you should also avoid all kinds of flour, baked foods, starchy vegetables, and sweet and juicy fruits.

In a nutshell, that means you should avoid:

- Baked goods like pastries, donuts, bread, cookies, pancakes, etc.
- All kinds of flours because even wholegrain flours are quickly converted into sugarPasta
- Most fruits
- Potatoes, especially fried potatoes
- All kinds of candy or chocolates
- Sweet soda and fruity drinks
- Canned foods
- Crackers
- Salad dressings
- Spreads and jams
- Dairy products
- Alcohol

☯ YOUR DIET SHOULD BE 80 PERCENT FRESH VEGETABLES, SEEDS, AND NUTS.

The remaining 20 percent should be cooked foods like red quinoa, whole grain barley, amaranth, millet, lentils, and beans. If you do not have a gluten or gliadin allergy or sensitivity, use whole grain spelt or kamut.

Cooking destroys the enzymes, which are needed to build healthy cells. When enzymes are heated to temperatures higher than 104° Fahrenheit or 40 Celsius, they are destroyed.

☯ YOU SHOULD AVOID ALL HYDROGENATED OILS AND TRANS FATS.

The best oils are cold pressed olive oil, walnut oil, and organic virgin coconut oil for cooking. The oils in avocados are also very healthy.

☯ YOU SHOULD AVOID MOST SEAFOOD.

Seafood is unfortunately loaded with toxins—especially lobsters, clams, and shrimp because they are responsible for cleaning the seabed and, therefore, are full of toxins. Tuna and all fish that are at the end of the food chain have a very high amount of mercury and should not be eaten. Currently, the only fish that can still be recommended is wild-caught salmon and other fast-growing, wild-caught fish.

☯ AVOID, IN GENERAL, ALL MANMADE FOOD.

It is full of preservatives, colors, MSG (monosodium glutamate food enhancer), sugar, hydrogenated fats, artificial sweeteners (Aspartame), GMO, etc.

If Mother Nature didn't make it, don't eat it.

❧ AVOID PESTICIDES AND CHEMICALS BY EATING ORGANIC FOOD.

If you cannot afford organic produce or it is not readily available in your area, don't use that as an excuse for not eating fresh vegetables. It is still better to eat fresh produce that has been chemically treated with pesticides than not to eat any vegetables at all.

❧ NO SOY PRODUCTS

Products such as soy sausages, meat, and soy milk are highly processed using many chemicals. Soy is also a phtyoestrogene and, therefore, contraindicated by all estrogen-related cancers, especially breast cancer.

Two glasses of soy milk per day for one month is enough to alter your menstrual cycle.

Infants fed soy formula consume an estimated five birth control pills' worth of estrogen every day.

❧ MOST CANCER PATIENTS SHOULD AVOID DAIRY PRODUCTS.

There is a high percentage of the population that is lactose intolerant; therefore, dairy products trigger allergies, inflammation, and weaken the immune system.

If you simply cannot live without dairy products, choose organic RAW milk and keep the amount to a minimum. Everything that is homogenized and pasteurized is considered toxic to your body. The molecular structure has been destroyed, making it no longer useful to your body.

☯ PROTEIN

Cancer patients need protein to protect them from cachexia.

The tumor itself consumes most of the energy; therefore, it is important to bring the overall energy of the patient up. There are many different opinions for obtaining good protein, and we believe it depends on personal choices too.

If protein is required to help a patient gain some energy, the items on the following list are suggested to be the best sources:

- Organic RAW eggs from grass-fed chickens (They taste very good in smoothies.)
- Organic rice protein, in powder form (Sun Warrior protein)
- Whey protein powder from an organic source (unless you are lactose intolerant)
- Hulled hemp seeds, which are very high in protein
- Beef from organic, grass-fed cows (small amounts)
- Wild-caught Alaskan salmon (small amounts)
- Cooked beans and legumes (on occasion)
- Spirulina (as much as you like)
- AlmondsSpinach, kale, and other vegetables (Eat mountains of vegetables.)

Protein is the most difficult nutrient to digest; therefore, the body needs most of its enzymes to break it down. If you add animal protein to your diet, it's important to supplement with additional enzymes. Otherwise the body has no enzymes left to destroy the cancer cells.

There is no doubt that we need protein, but for a cancer patient it should be easy to digest. Eggs, which contain all necessary amino acids, are viewed as a complete protein. They are, in their raw form, the easiest to be broken down by the body's enzymes.

Beef and salmon should be eaten only in very small quantities (once or twice per week in tiny quantities if at all). During the initial healing phase, we suggest patients completely refrain from eating these proteins until the body is stronger.

The best plan is to eat protein in the morning (a protein smoothie) until 1 p.m. Then the body has enough time to produce enzymes to deal with the tumor and the protein meal the next day.

☯ FRESH, ORGANIC, GREEN VEGETABLE JUICES

They are the best cancer-fighting foods. They detox and alkaline the body. You can have as much as you like and the more the better. Look up the Gerson Protocol as it uses juicing as a healing element.

☯ AVOID COFFEE AND CAFFEINE ENERGY DRINKS

Coffee is very acidic and adds to the acidic environment in which the cancer cells thrive and grow.

☯ GREEN TEA

Green tea is a much better alternative to any drink as it has anti-angiogenesis properties.

☯ DRINK LOTS OF WATER

Drink half of your body weight in ounces. The water needs to be of good quality—free of chlorine, fluoride, and chemicals. Spring water is a good source. On the website http://www.findaspring.com/ you can find sources where you can bottle your spring water at a very affordable price. Don't buy spring water in soft plastic bottles which contain BPA or the hard plastic refill bottles as they contain BPA too. It is best to fill up your water yourself and use a glass container.

There are also very good water filters on the market that you can install in your home. If your water is fluoridated, you need to buy a reverse osmosis filter with a mineralization cartridge to reactivate, mineralize, and oxygenate the water. No other filter can effectively remove the fluoride. No matter what they tell you, don't believe it. If your water supply comes from a tank, you have many more options.

☯ HEALTHY ALTERNATIVES TO SUGAR

Stevia is a sweet-tasting herb native to South and Central America and is known for its sweet taste. Stevia does not trigger an insulin response (Glycemic index of zero) and is, therefore, safe to use. It has virtually no calories and is 200 to 300 times sweeter than real sugar. There are many different brands out there; from NOW ON, look for a pure one like Stevita® or Stevia. Sample the options and find the one you like best. You should still use these sweeteners sparingly; the more you tone down your sweet tooth, the better.

Xylitol, which comes from birch trees, has been used as a sweetening agent in food since the 1960s. It is even produced by your body during normal metabolism. Xylitol (Glycemic index of 7) has the same sweetness as sucrose, but it is clearly healthier. Xylitol is currently used in chewing gum, gumdrops, and hard candy. It is low in calories and has no unpleasant aftertaste. Extremely large amounts may produce weight gain, diarrhea, or cause dysfunction in some organs. So please be cautious with your consumption. It's not a substitute to be abused.

Yakon Syrup is made from a Peruvian or Mexican root vegetable. The substance fructo-oligo-saccharides, which causes the root to be sweet, actually feeds the good bacteria in the intestines but does not cause the undesirable blood sugar response in the body. Only use this substitute occasionally and in small amounts.

Unfortunately, **agave nectar** is not as good as it is proclaimed to be as it is composed of 50 to 65 percent fructose. Fructose is the main culprit in feeding cancer cells.

☯ MUST AVOID FRUCTOSE

So what kind of fruit and how much are we allowed to eat? To be on the safe side, we should not eat more than 15 grams of fructose per day. Below is a table taken from the book *The Sugar Fix* by Dr. Richard Johnson.

If you are interested, watch this video of Dr. Johnson on YouTube:

"Sugar: The Bitter Truth"
http://www.youtube.com/watch?v=dBnniua6-oM

Fruit	Serving Size	Grams of Fructose
Limes	1 medium	0
Lemons	1 medium	0.6
Cranberries	1 cup	0.7
Passion fruit	1 medium	0.9
Prune	1 medium	1.2
Apricot	1 medium	1.3
Guava	2 medium	2.2
Date (Deglet Noor style)	1 medium	2.6
Cantaloupe	1/8 of med. melon	2.8
Raspberries	1 cup	3.0
Clementine	1 medium	3.4
Kiwifruit	1 medium	3.4
Blackberries	1 cup	3.5
Star fruit	1 medium	3.6
Cherries, sweet	10	3.8
Strawberries	1 cup	3.8
Cherries, sour	1 cup	4.0
Pineapple	1 slice (3.5" x .75")	4.0

Grapefruit, pink or red	1/2 medium	4.3
Boysenberries	1 cup	4.6
Tangerine/mandarin orange	1 medium	4.8
Nectarine	1 medium	5.4
Peach	1 medium	5.9
Orange (navel)	1 medium	6.1
Papaya	1/2 medium	6.3
Honeydew	1/8 of med. melon	6.7
Banana	1 medium	7.1
Blueberries	1 cup	7.4
Date (Medjool)	1 medium	7.7
Apple (composite)	1 medium	9.5
Persimmon	1 medium	10.6
Watermelon	1/16 med. melon	11.3
Pear	1 medium	11.8
Raisins	1/4 cup	12.3
Grapes, seedless (green or red)	1 cup	12.4
Mango	1/2 medium	16.2
Apricots, dried	1 cup	16.4
Figs, dried	1 cup	23.0

☯ CANCER-FIGHTING FOODS

- Dark green, leafy vegetables
- Flaxseed oil and cod liver oil
- Cruciferous vegetables
- Almonds
- Brazil nuts
- Sweet potatoes
- Kelp

☯ SUPER FOODS

Maca powder: Is a root vegetable rich in minerals such as calcium, magnesium, potassium, sulfur, iron, and silica. It contains nearly 20 amino acids, including seven essential amino acids. Maca helps stabilize and maintain many of the body's systems such as the endocrine, circulatory, and immune systems.

Goji berries: Are packed with vitamins, minerals, protein, and antioxidants.

Acai berries: Deliver powerful antioxidants, essential fatty acids, fiber, and amino acids.

Spirulina: Is an excellent source of protein, chlorophyll, trace minerals, vitamins and antioxidants. Spirulina balances the pH of the body and protects against radioactive particles. Spirulina has nature's highest source of vitamin B12. Spirulina raises glutathione and therefore reduces liver and kidney toxicity.

Chlorella: Contains an abundance of chlorophyll. Chlorella can help strengthen our immune system; it is alkaline-forming and detoxifying.

Aloe vera: The gel of raw aloe vera contains vitamins C and E, plus the minerals calcium, magnesium, zinc, selenium, and chromium, as well as antioxidants, fiber, amino acids, enzymes, sterols, and lignins, and, most importantly, polysaccharides. It is the polysaccharides in aloe that help it do everything from fighting infections to boosting the immune system.

Wheat grass juice: Contains bioavailable chlorophyll, many amino acids, choline, magnesium, and potassium. The juice strengthens the cell, increases blood alkaline, detoxifies the liver and blood stream, and chemically neutralizes the polluting elements in our environment.

Hemp seed: Contains all of the necessary essential fatty acids in the perfect ratio absorption. It also contains 34 percent protein and all 20 of the known amino acids. It is high in fiber and contains antioxidants such as vitamin E and vitamin A, other vitamins, minerals, trace minerals, and even chlorophyll.

☯ ALKALINE FOODS

Cancer cells thrive in an acidic environment because of their shortened metabolism. All healthy cells are somewhat paralyzed in an acidic milieu and can't perform their duties. Therefore, your immune system will not be fully operational if you are not changing the pH to alkaline. You can purchase pH test strips at the pharmacy, or you can even find them at places where you find swimming pool or fish aquarium supplies. Obviously, the Internet is another option for ordering them.

The second urine of the morning should be used to accurately test your pH, or you can use saliva, but you must first spit, discarding all of the saliva from your mouth before you do the test.

Many foods will help you achieve an optimal pH level in your body. The culprits of an acidic pH in the first place are sugar, baked goods, large amounts of meat, sodas, coffee, etc.

Below is a list for alkaline forming foods:

- Garlic
- Asparagus
- Watercress
- Beets
- Broccoli
- Brussels sprouts
- Cabbage
- Carrots
- Cauliflower
- Celery
- Chard
- Chlorella
- Collard greens
- Cucumbers
- Eggplants

- Kale
- Kohlrabi
- Lettuce
- Mushrooms
- Mustard greens
- Dilce
- Dandelions
- Onions
- Peas
- Peppers
- Sea veggies
- Spirulina
- Sprouts
- Alfalfa barley grass
- Wheat grass
- Wild greens
- Almonds
- Fermented Tempeh
- Herbs

☯ MEAL REPLACEMENTS

If there is any reason you cannot eat a normal meal anymore and need to be fed with liquid formulas, then here is a list of the best meal replacement formulas available at the moment:

· http://www.livingfuel.com/LivingFuel_Products.aspx

LivingFuel is offering different products that you just mix with water.

· http://theultimatelife.net/CatalogMeal.htm

· The Ultimate Meal is free of yeast-based vitamins and minerals, soy protein, MSG, salt, wheat, corn, yeast, eggs, dairy products, sugar, honey, fructose, caffeine, ginseng, etc. It also has no artificial preservatives, flavors, coloring, fillers or animal products.

· http://www.gardenoflife.com/

Garden of Life is offering different products as organic Raw Protein, Raw Meal (organic raw meal replacement), Perfect Food.

Famous Cancer protocols

☯ BUDWIG DIET:

The famous Budwig diet consists of combining flaxseed oil and cottage cheese/quark. Dr. Budwig found that this combination promotes bio-oxygenation and also changes the oil to a water-soluble form, which makes it absorbable for the body.

The Budwig Protocol incorporated not only her flaxseed oil and cottage muesli but also a strict diet regime. Unfortunately, many patients do not strictly follow the program; therefore, they are not successful in treating their cancer.

The Budwig Cancer Center in Spain was directly authorized by Dr. Johanna Budwig to continue with her treatments. The Center teaches her diet approach as the basis of their program.

As cancers are much more aggressive today, they require additional measures to fight it; therefore, patients in their center receive multiple treatments.

These treatments include supplementation, far-infrared sauna, exercise, PEMF, detoxification, addressing microbes, parasites, candida, pancreatic enzymes, sodium bicarbonate/DMSO, tumor control, hyperthermia, reflexology, natural oxygen therapies, lymph drainage, and more.

The Body-Mind Connection is very well addressed here too.

To get in contact with Dr. Lyold Jenkins and receive a "no obligation" health diagnosis, simply contact Dr. Jenkins at BudwigCenter@gmail.com.

☯ THE GERSON PROTOCOL

The Gerson protocol should be the basis of all cancer treatments.

With its whole-body approach to healing, the Gerson Therapy naturally reactivates your body's magnificent ability to heal itself-- with no damaging side-effects. Over 200 articles in respected medical literature and thousands of people cured of their "incurable" diseases document the Gerson Therapy's effectiveness. The Gerson Therapy is one of the few treatments to have a 60-year history of success.

The Gerson Therapy is a powerful, natural treatment that boosts your body's own immune system to heal cancer, arthritis, heart disease, allergies, and many other degenerative diseases. One aspect of the Gerson Therapy that sets it apart from most other treatment methods is its all-encompassing nature. An abundance of nutrients from 13 fresh, organic juices are consumed every day, providing your body with a super-dose of enzymes, minerals, and nutrients. These substances then break down diseased tissue in the body, while enemas aid in eliminating the lifelong buildup of toxins from the liver.

Throughout our lives our bodies are being filled with a variety of disease and cancer-causing pollutants. These toxins reach us through the air we breathe, the food we eat, the medicines we take, and the water we drink. As more of these poisons are used every day and cancer rates continue to climb, being able to turn to a proven, natural, detoxifying treatment like the Gerson Therapy is not only reassuring, but necessary.

Although its philosophy of cleansing and reactivating the body is simple, the Gerson Therapy is a complex method of treatment requiring significant attention to detail. While many patients have made full recoveries practicing the Gerson Therapy on their own, for best results we encourage starting treatment at a licensed Gerson treatment center.

The Gerson Therapy seeks to regenerate the body to health, supporting each important metabolic requirement by flooding the body with nutrients from almost 20 pounds of organically grown fruits and vegetables daily. Most are used to make fresh raw juice, which should be consumed by one glass every hour, 13 times per day. Raw and cooked solid foods are generously consumed. Oxygenation is usually more than doubled as oxygen deficiency in the blood contributes to many degenerative diseases. The metabolism is also stimulated through the addition of thyroid, potassium, and other supplements, and by avoiding heavy animal fats, excess protein, sodium, and other toxins.

You will find all the information about the Gerson protocol at http://gerson.org/.

Please understand that this list of diet recommendations is not complete. A complete guide would be a very big book! Also, diet is determined on an individual basis and depends on the person and his or her physical condition. Many clinics incorporate a metabolic testing, blood type, and consideration of hereditary issues to find your perfect diet, and it is always important to see how well you feel with what you eat. If you get weak and lose energy and muscle mass, then it's certainly worth considering a change.

Let us repeat . . . NO diet fits all!

Some people have a very weak digestive system due to disease and drugs. They won't be able to tolerate an 80 percent raw diet right from the beginning. These patients need to take it slowly, one step at a time!Excluding all sugars and manmade products is already a huge step towards good health. Don't forget, we are what we eat!!

> *Each patient carries his own doctor inside him.*
>
> *-Albert Schweitzer*

Supplementation

Supplements are meant to support the body in its innate ability to heal. They support the immune system, the liver, and kidneys and fill the body up with the nutrients of which it is deprived. Through toxins, bad eating habits, lifestyle, and other factors, your body is deficient in many nutrients. Taking these nutrients, in addition to eating a healthy diet and making various lifestyle changes, will help you combat disease.

Supplements are not a substitute for a bad diet!!!

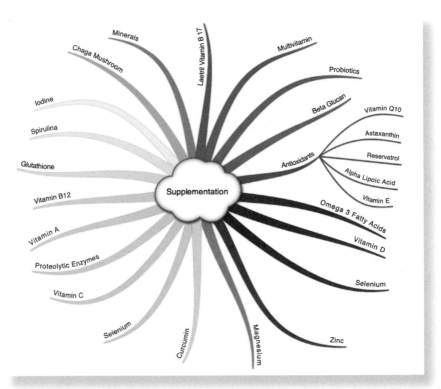

Believe me, supplements won't help compensate for a diet of junk food and toxic food. Food is still the #1 method for obtaining the nutrients your body needs. For example, broccoli not only includes Lutein-zeaxanthin, but over 590 other vital elements. So, if you take a supplement, you might get a boost in lutein, but you will miss out on all the other minerals, vitamins, and vital nutrients.

That's another reason you must consider the quality of the supplements. The more natural and unprocessed the supplement, the better it is. This is best illustrated by the Gerson protocol—you just juice mountains of vegetables and drink the juice. This provides everything in its original form, and your body heals.

Finding good supplements is not an easy task as the market is flooded with bad and cheap hoaxes. You can buy absolutely worthless synthetic supplements in supermarkets and food chains, which will cause more harm than good.

So how do you find good ones? What do you look out for?

Most prescription **vitamin D** is vitamin D2 (ergocalciferol) which is less effective than vitamin D3 (cholecalciferol). Vitamin D2 is the synthetic version and vitamin D3 is the natural one—and identical to the one our body produces when exposed to sunshine.ALL supplements need to be free of dairy, soy, non-GMO, corn, wheat, gluten, colors, fillers, artificial flavors, etc.

To get the maximum benefit, **vitamin E** should always be consumed in the form of mixed natural tocopherols and tocotrienols. Natural vitamin E is always listed as the "d-" form (d-alpha-tocopherol, d-beta-tocopherol, d-gamma-tocopherol, d-delta-tocopherol). The synthetic vitamin E is listed as "dl-" forms (d-alpha-tocopheryl succinate, for example).

You always want a good balance among calcium, magnesium, and potassium.

The **multivitamin** must go way beyond RDA (Recommended Daily Allowance) and RDI (Recommended Daily Intake) guidelines as they definitely define the absolute lowest amount of intake.

Do not believe that you can pack all vitamins and minerals into a one-serving-size pill per day. The majority of your vitamin intake should come from nutrients in natural food sources (vegetables, fruits and herbs).

Vitamin B12 should never be made out of Cyanocobalamin as this is the synthetic form and actually turns into a toxic, poisonous cyanide molecule. It is cheap and, therefore, is used in many supplements. It should be from the natural form, Methylcobolamin. It is also pre-methylated, meaning it's ready for your biochemistry to put to immediate use. The preferred method for taking Vitamin B12 successfully is by injections, sublingual absorption, and skin absorption.

Omega-3 oil should contain the omega-3 fats EPA and DHA and not the plant-based omega-3 fat ALA, which is only converted in small amounts to EPA and DHA in your body. ALA is contained in nuts, seeds, and flaxseed oil. It is also important to make sure that any fish consumed are naturally harvested from unpolluted waters and are not farmed. The oils should be extracted without the use of chemicals. The fish oil should be independently tested for heavy metals like mercury, lead, cadmium, PCBs, etc.

Some important facts about a **probiotic supplement** are that it shows high potency through independent lab tests. It needs to be high in Lactobacillus acidophilus, and its count needs to be in the billions. IT SHOULD also BE free of dairy, soy, corn, wheat, gluten, and GMO.

When choosing a **whey powder**, you should look out for several important factors. The whey powder should come from cows, which are raised free range, pasture-grazed, grass-fed, and not treated with synthetic growth hormones (rBGH). It also should be free of artificial additives, flavors, colors, preservatives, GMO ingredients, pesticides, herbicides, and artificial sweeteners.

Do not use the whey protein isolate as your body cannot assimilate proteins in isolated form. Isolates are caused by over-processing deficiencies in key amino-acids and nutritional cofactors. Buy the whey protein concentrate!

The following recommended supplements are based on a summary of interviews we conducted of all of the doctors during our journey. It is not complete, and none of the supplements should be taken without the consultation of a qualified doctor, nutritionist, or naturopathic doctor.

David Getoff made a very good DVD about "Supplementation." His step-by-step process is very empowering.   http://www. canceriscurablenow.tv/product/nutritional-supplements-dvd

> *Never forget that if a nutritional product or food (or, as far as I am concerned, any drug) makes you feel bad, you should reduce the dose or stop using the product. Substances that are supportive to your body will not generally produce any undesirable "symptoms" if taken at the proper dose for your body.*
>
> *-David Getoff, ND, CCN, CTN, FAAIM*

A while ago, we were asked to sample a particular green powder to determine if we would like to promote it in our list. But after testing it, we decided not to do so as our whole family reacted with nausea, illness, allergies, and so on. Who would think that a garden green powder could do that?

Kinesiology is a great way to test supplements to see if you agree with them or not. It's vital, and most of the doctors we have worked with use it. We advise you to do the same—either with a partner, friend, or with a physician. Doctors often use energetic testing; the ELISA and EAV testing are recommended.

http://www.youtube.com/watch?v=2q9JTWEz8Fc&feature=related

☯ VITAMIN D / SUNLIGHT

Yes, we need sunshine and NO! **Sunshine does not cause cancer**. Without sunshine there would be no life on earth. Plants produce energy through sunshine. It is this energy that we need to survive.

Research indicates that vitamin D, whether produced in the skin through exposure to the sun or taken as a supplement, helps cancer patients.

If you search the US National Institutes of Health's Medline online database for "cancer vitamin D," you will find over 5,000 papers, some dating back nearly 60 years.

> *Michael Holick, MD, Boston University, professor of medicine, has come right out and said it, "We can reduce cancer risk by 30 to 50 percent by increasing Vitamin D.*
>
> *"Dr. Cedric Garland of the UC San Diego School of Medicine and Moore's Cancer Center published a paper saying that the risk of breast cancer could be cut by 50 percent if people had vitamin D serum levels somewhere between 40 to 50 nanograms per milliliter.*

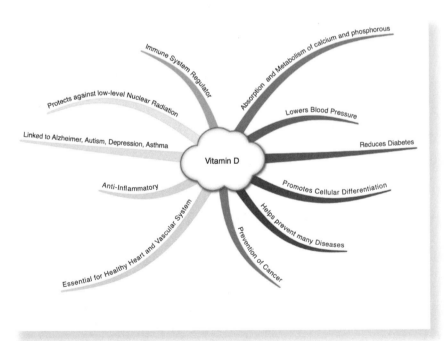

Our body cannot produce vitamin D without sunshine.

Vitamin D is very important:

- It produces healthy bones.

- It helps prevent at least 16 different types of cancer including pancreatic, lung, ovarian, prostate, and skin cancers.

- It is essential for a healthy heart and vascular system.

- It reduces diabetes.

- It is linked to Alzheimer's, autism, depression, asthma and many more.

Unfortunately, the average person is not getting enough sunshine anymore because of our lifestyles—we spend most of the day indoors. When we do get out into the sun, we are mostly covered with clothes, or our exposed skin is covered with sunscreen.

Studies are showing that most of us are vitamin D deficient.

Normal sunscreen, available in every supermarket or drug store, is filled with cancer-causing ingredients and adds to the risk of getting cancer. There are many natural and organic sun creams available that can be used when someone needs to be in the sun for a prolonged period of time.

Some very good brands are:

- UV Natural Sunscreen SPF30+

- Badger, All Natural Sunscreen, SPF 30, Unscented

- Soleo Organics all natural SUNSCREEN, SPF 30

The daily recommended intake of a vitamin D3 supplement is only 600 IU/day, but researchers have found that a daily intake of 4,000-8,000 IU/day are absolutely needed to maintain blood levels of vitamin D metabolites to reduce the risk of cancer by half.

The "normal" 25-hydroxy vitamin D lab range is between 20-56 ng/ml, but your vitamin D level should never be below 32 ng/ml. Any levels below 20 ng/ml are considered seriously deficient, increasing your risk of getting as many as 16 different cancers and autoimmune diseases such as multiple sclerosis and rheumatoid arthritis.

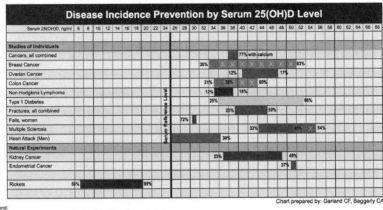

The OPTIMAL value that you're looking for is 50-70 ng/ml (or 125-175 nmol/L).

This range applies to everyone: children, adolescents, adults, and seniors.

(http://articles.mercola.com/sites/articles/archive/2009/10/10/vitamin-d-experts-reveal-the-truth.aspx)

It is very important that you watch the YouTube video by Carole A. Baggerly uploaded by the University of California and the website she created with her husband.

http://www.grassrootshealth.net/ a public Health Promotion Organization

http://www.youtube.com/watch?v=TQ-qekFoi-o&feature=relmfu

☯ MULTI VITAMIN

There are many good products to choose from, and the ones listed here should help you compare them and to know what to look for. All of them, in our opinion, are well put together and have sufficient amounts of the individual substances.

> *The secret is in getting your body so chemically unloaded and nutrient primed, that it heals itself.*
>
> *- Dr. Sherry Rogers*

Perfect Blend (standard or iron free) from SuperNutrition

Beyond Chelation Improved from Longevity Plus

Dr. Mercola Multivitamin Plus (Whole Food + Vital Minerals)

Daily Advantage from Dr. Williams www.drdavidwilliams.com

(Recommended by Dr. Garry Gordon, Bill Henderson and David Getoff; all featured in our movie)

☯ MINERALS AND TRACE MINERALS

Minerals and trace minerals are essential for our body to function properly. They are needed in all bodily functions as activators and catalysts for other nutrients and vitamins. They are the building blocks of enzymes, hormones, and other natural body chemicals, balancing body fluids with pressure and are essential in digestion and absorption of nutrients by our body.

A loss of equilibrium causes cells to burst, nervous disorders, brain damage, and excessive growth. In regards to the alkaline—acid-balanced cancer can be caused by the acidification of the blood, lymph, and all cellular tissues.

Quinton Marine Plasma is, by far, one of the best sources and should be taken daily.

☯ VITAMIN A

Vitamin A is found in animal sources such as liver, fish oils, egg yolks, and dairy products.

Vitamin A

- Prevents night blindness and eye disorders
- Enhances immunity
- Is important for formation of bones and teeth
- Aids in fat storage
- Protects against colds, flu, and infections of kidneys, bladder, lungs, and mucous membranesIs an antioxidant
- Helps to protect against cancer
- Lowers cholesterol levels
- Guards against heart disease and stroke
- Is needed for utilization of protein

Doctors' experience and clinical evidence both show that vitamin A helps prevent cancer. This has been known for a long time. "The association of vitamin A and cancer was initially reported in 1926 when rats, fed a vitamin A-deficient diet, developed gastric carcinomas."

The NIH (National Institutes of Health) says, "Dietary intake studies suggest an association between diets rich in beta-carotene and vitamin A and a lower risk of many types of cancer."

A great article to read in regards to vitamin A is the following:

http://www.orthomolecular.org/resources/omns/v04n09.shtml

Taking large amounts of vitamin A—100,000 international units per day—over a long period of time, can be toxic to the liver.

David Getoff prescribes 20-30,000iu of vitamin A per day unless overdose symptoms develop; in which case, he reduces the dose. He has only had one incidence of overdose in the past 20 years. As soon as the patient is taken off of the high dose, the symptoms disappear without any damage to the body.

☯ VITAMIN B12

Vitamin B12 is found almost exclusively in animal tissue. A vitamin B12 deficiency can be caused by a strict vegetarian diet and can be found in people with digestive disorders.

Vitamin B12 is needed to prevent anemia, aids folic acid in regulating the formation of red blood cells, and helps in the utilization of iron.

But there are many more functions that require vitamin B12:

- Proper digestion
- Absorption of nutrients
- Synthesis of proteins
- Metabolism of carbohydrates and fats
- Prevents nerve damage
- Maintains fertility
- Promotes normal growth
- Enhances sleep patterns
- Tissue and cellular repair
- DNA synthesis

Vitamin B12 can be stored in the body and deficiency symptoms can take three to six years to develop.

Blood tests can easily reveal if a deficiency exists:

- CBC (Complete Blood Count): A group of tests ordered routinely to screen for blood cell abnormalities. It measures cell types, quantities, and characteristics. With both B12 and folate deficiencies, the amount of hemoglobin and RBC count may be low, and the RBCs are abnormally large (macrocytic or megaloblastic), resulting in anemia. White blood cells and platelets also may be decreased.

- Homocysteine levels may be elevated in both B12 and folate deficiency.

As mentioned before, vitamin B12 should be taken in the form of sublingual tablets, spray, or by injection. Please look out for the natural form of vitamin B12, Methylcobolamin.

☯ ANTIOXIDANTS

Antioxidants are molecules that act as the body's first line of defense against damage from a natural process called oxidation. They destroy substances called free radicals, which occur naturally in our body and are also left behind by smog, cigarette smoke, radiation, and toxins. The best antioxidants you can get are the ones in your food. They are in all vegetables—especially in green, fresh, organically grown ones.

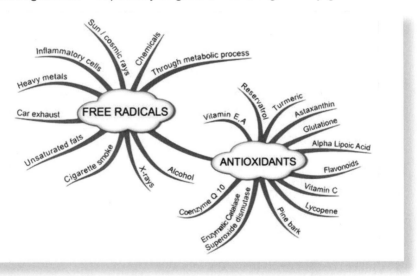

Vitamin Q10 is an antioxidant and is synthesized within the body but not always in sufficient amounts. Vitamin Q10 is involved in energy production in the cells and boosts the immune system that is highly energy-dependent. Several studies have documented an immune-enhancing effect of Q10 and a benefit in cancer patients.

Astaxanthin is a powerful antioxidant, and the best one is extracted from marine algae. It potentially reduces DNA damage caused by free radicals.

Resveratrol is found in red wine because of the content of grape seeds and grape skins. Researchers have found anti-cancer and immune-stimulating effects with resveratrol. It has been shown to induce apoptotic cell death in human leukemia cells as well as in some breast carcinoma cells.

A large concentration is needed to have any health benefits. It is not possible to obtain this level of resveratrol by drinking wine. It is best to use a more potent form of supplement.

Alpha Lipoic Acid has been called the "universal" antioxidant because it boosts glutathione levels in cells and has potent antioxidant actions. It also has a metal-chelating ability, helping the body rid itself of accumulated ingested toxins.

Vitamin E is an antioxidant that is important in the prevention of cancer and cardiovascular disease.

It also:

- Promotes normal blood clotting and healing
- Prevents cell damage
- Reduces blood pressure
- Maintains healthy nerves and muscles
- Strengthens capillary walls
- Promotes healthy skin and hair
- Is successful in treating fatty liverThe natural form of vitamin E is far more active than the synthetic form. As mentioned in the beginning of the chapter, you should read the labels of your supplement product and buy only the d-alph-tocopherol form.

☯ PROTEOLYTIC ENZYMES

Dr. Constantine Kotsanis, MD, says:" I find that cancer patients who do enzyme therapy have better treatment outcomes."

Scientific research and evidence show that enzymes break up blood cell clumps; thin the blood; break down carbohydrates, fats, and proteins; rebalance inflammatory responses; promote a strong immune system; promote healthy joints; and control cancer growth.

One hundred years ago, Dr. Beard's theory explained that misplaced trophoblasts, what we today call stem cells, are the source of cancer.

Pancreatic enzymes control placental growth and, because cancer cells result from misplaced placental cells, pancreatic enzymes also control cancer cell growth.

"At least 86 percent of all cancer conditions could be adequately treated and/or prevented by diet and pancreatic enzymes. Cancer is a symptom of inadequate and deficient protein metabolism. The real problem is protein metabolism, not cancer," says Dr. Kelly.

Many doctors around the world today treat cancer using high proteolytic enzyme therapy.

Wobenzym N, a proteolytic enzyme supplement from Europe, is documented to lower C-reactive protein levels of 30 percent.

C-reactive protein is the marker for chronic inflammation. These results will without doubt help every cancer patient in his healing process.

Dr. Gonzalez, a New York-based immunologist, has developed a cancer treatment regimen that incorporates diet, nutritional supplements, and detoxification. Every cancer patient on his regimen consumes between 130-175 capsules each day. The supplements include a range of vitamins, minerals, trace elements, anti-oxidants, and animal glandular products; they are prescribed according to the patient's need. In addition to these supplements, every patient takes large quantities of pancreas product (proteolytic enzymes), which provide the main anti-cancer action, in Dr. Gonzalez's opinion.

Dr. Gonzalez's protocol is based on the research of Dr. Beard (the enzyme therapy of cancer and its scientific basis). Articles about his scientific efforts have been published in conventional, peer-reviewed literature.

☯ PROBIOTICS

Probiotics are very important to support your good and friendly bacteria living in your gut. These so-called friendly bacteria assist with digestion, keeping other harmful bacteria at bay and stimulating the immune system.

Total health begins in your gut.

Because we consume so many antibiotics—even without being on an antibiotic treatment—our intestinal bacteria growth is extremely diminished.

Why is it so important?

Because it houses the majority of the human immune system; approximately 70 percent of it is located in the gastro-intestinal tract.

Healthy gut flora populations protect against invading microbes simply by taking up space and by being generally more proficient at obtaining nutrients than the intruders.

Intestinal flora can even influence the growth and formation of organs crucial to proper immune function. Take the thymus, for example, the primary function of which is to produce T-lymphocytes, also known as T-cells. T-cells are a type of white blood cells that have two functions. Killer T-cells destroy the body's own cells that have been infected by viruses or bacteria; this prevents the offending microbe from replicating and causing more damage. Helper T-cells stimulate the production of antibodies. Both are vital, and both are made possible by the thymus. The thymus, in turn, is dependent on intestinal flora.

☯ ZINC

Zinc is an essential mineral found in every cell in the body. It stimulates the activity of over 100 enzymes.

Some of its known functions are as follow:

- Detoxifies lead, mercury, and cadmium
- Maintains a healthy immune system
- Accelerates wound healing
- Reduces colds
- Maintains sense of taste and smell
- Synthesizes DNA
- Maintains sight
- Helps sperm develop
- Promotes ovulation and fertilization
- Protects against prostate problems
- Helps protect against cancer

New developments in zinc research have yielded some amazing findings. The latest research shows that zinc can protect against esophageal cancer.

Zinc not only improves cell-mediated immune reactions but also functions as an antioxidant and anti-inflammatory agent. Oxidative stress and chronic inflammation have been implicated in the development of many cancers. Research shows that nearly 65 percent of patients with head and neck cancer were zinc-deficient, based on their cellular zinc concentrations. (Pub Med study, "Zinc in Cancer Prevention")

Zinc and selenium are two very important minerals that should be integrated into every cancer protocol.

☯ SELENIUM

The mineral selenium has been shown in multiple studies to be an effective tool in warding off various types of cancer, including breast, esophageal, stomach, prostate, liver, and bladder cancers.

Selenium, especially in combination with vitamin D, vitamin C and vitamin E, has strong cancer-fighting properties. Countries like Australia are very deficient in the mineral selenium in their soil; therefore, a deficiency exists in the food grown there. In that case, it is very important to supplement. The recommended dose is 200 micrograms a day.

Brazil nuts are very high in selenium.

Selenium protects the immune system by preventing the formation of free radicals that can damage the body. It also helps to stop damaged cells from reproducing and, therefore, directly helps to avoid the growth of cancer.

☯ VITAMIN C

Vitamin C is one of the most important vitamins for any cancer patient.

Benefits of vitamin C:

- Induction of apoptosis and cell death mechanisms
- Improved immune surveillance and tumor recognition
- Anti-inflammatory
- Strong antioxidant
- Immune stimulation
- Detoxifier
- Increase absorption of nutrients
- Provides energy in cellular chemistry

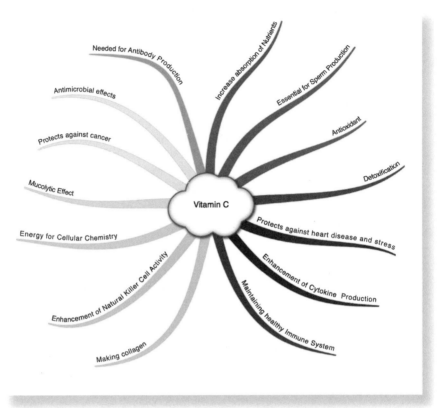

Needed for Antibody Production

Antimicrobial effects

Protects against cancer

Mucolytic Effect

Energy for Cellular Chemistry

Enhancement of Natural Killer Cell Activity

Making collagen

Increase absorption of Nutrients

Essential for Sperm Production

Antioxidant

Detoxification

Vitamin C

Protects against heart disease and stress

Enhancement of Cytokine Production

Maintaining healthy Immune System

Therapeutic doses for the treatment of cancer or degenerative diseases can only be achieved intravenously by giving IV vitamin C blood concentrations 200 times higher than possible through oral dosing. This is based on the work of Dr. Linus Pauling, winner of the Nobel Prize for chemistry in1954 and for peace in 1963.

Small amounts (25 grams) of vitamin C, two or three times a week, can be life-saving to a cancer patient if properly administered intravenously.

Vitamin C is water-soluble and not stored in the body, so it is crucial to constantly take oral vitamin C to maximize immune function and overcome infections.

"Infections depress levels of vitamin B6 and vitamin C. The right dose of vitamin C will stop every infection in its track without needing to use antibiotics," says Dr. Garry Gordon.

The best vitamin C that can be taken orally is BioNRgyC. This vitamin C can be taken two to three times a day, at a dose of 1 rounded teaspoon in some water without any stomach upset. (1 rounded teaspoon =4,000mg)

(Recommended by David Getoff, Dr. Garry Gordon, and Dr. Conneally, all featured in our movie.)

Why is vitamin C so important for detoxification? Because every time it leaves the body, it takes toxins with it. It is this reason that vitamin C is called the poor man's chelator. It is necessary to maintain high levels of vitamin C in the blood 24/7. This can be tested with VitaChek C Stix. When the stick turns from green to the brightest yellow possible, you have achieved a high saturation of vitamin C.

http://www.naturalhealthyconcepts.com/vita-chek-C-50.html

☯ OMEGA 3

There are two basic categories of essential fatty acids, omega-3 (DHA and EPA) and omega-6, based on their chemical structure. Omega-3 oil can be obtained through fish and krill oil. Most people are dangerously deficient in omega-3 oils from marine life. The typical Western diet is high in saturated fats from meat products and very low in omega-3 fish oils. Vegetarian diets tend to be low in DHA and EPA too as these essential fatty acids are not available in vegetables. Vegetarians must rely on their body's limited ability to convert ALA (alpha linolenic acid found in flaxoil and soyoil) into DHA and EPA.

Because of their unique structure, DHA and EPA have unique functions within our body. Both are involved in a healthy cardiovascular system, immune processes, and help form healthy prostaglandins.

Omega-3 benefits:

- Fight depression

- Fight inflammatory disease
- Cardiovascular health
- Immune system health
- Brain and nerve function
- Eye and vision health
- Joint health

When choosing a high quality fish oil, it is important to make sure that the fish source delivers a high content of EPA and DHA. The production process must retain the vital nutrients, provide antioxidant nutrients for preservation, and provide free radical protection. We must also be certain that only toxin-free fish are used—free of mercury, PCBs, heavy metals, and other toxins.

☯ IODINE

Iodine is detected in every organ and tissue in the body. Iodine is absolutely necessary for a healthy thyroid as well as healthy ovaries, breasts, and prostate.

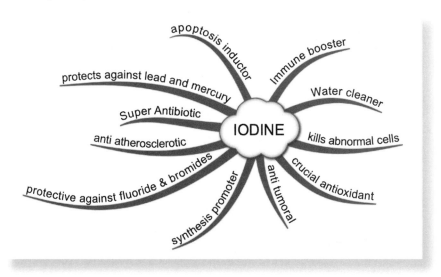

When dealing with toxic chemicals every day, it is important to have iodine as a protective agent against several common poisons like fluoride, bromide, and also to help eliminate lead and mercury.

Iodine is a crucial antioxidant and apoptosis inductor (programmed cell death) with anti-tumoral and anti-atherosclerotic activity. Iodine kills abnormal cells floating in the body.

In a study of 60 cancer sufferers, all 60, which means 100 percent, were seriously deficient in iodine. I assure you the problem is population-wide, writes Dr. Robert Rowen.

Breast tissue has an affinity for iodine. Iodine deficiency causes fibrocystic breast disease with nodules, cyst enlargement, pain, and scar tissue. Adequate tissue iodine helps guide estrogen into friendly pathways that support the proper functioning of female sex hormones.

Along with magnesium and selenium, iodine is one of the most deficient minerals in our body.

Iodine and selenium are required for the synthesis of thyroid hormones.

Symptoms of iodine deficiency are:

- Muscle cramps
- Cold hands and feetProneness to weight gain
- Poor memory
- Constipation
- Depression
- Headaches
- Edema
- Myalgia
- Weakness
- Dry skin
- Brittle nails

Iodine can be found in food such as (most) sea foods, unrefined sea salt, kelp and other seaweeds, butter, pineapple, artichokes, asparagus, dark green vegetables, and eggs.

The recommended supplement by Dr. Mark Sircus is nascent iodine.

As iodine is a strong chelator, start with a small amount to keep detoxification symptoms low.

One drop of nascent iodine is 0.2 mg.

For additional energy and general improved health, take five drops daily.

If recommended by your healthcare professional for assistance with a chronic health concern, take five drops four times a day. Always take on empty stomach.

Please consult a health care provider before taking iodine.

☯ MAGNESIUM

Magnesium deficiencies are one of the most common nutritional problems. A low level of magnesium makes nearly every disease worse.

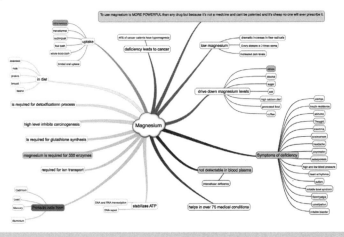

- Magnesium is the single most important mineral for maintaining proper electrical balance and facilitating smooth metabolism in the cells.

- Magnesium protects the cell against oxyradical damage, assists in the absorption and metabolism of B vitamins, as well as vitamins C and E.

- Magnesium protects the brain from the toxic effects of chemicals and is associated with glutathione production.

- Magnesium is a vital catalyst in enzyme activity, especially for those involved in energy production.

- A healthy immune system is driven by white blood cells that require good magnesium levels.

- Magnesium is directly linked to the body's production of DHEA, often called the "Feel Good Hormone." DHEA levels dramatically decline with age.

- It can reduce fatigue and stress and is a component of every healthy muscle cell.

- Magnesium stabilizes ATP and enables DNA and RNA transcription and repair.

It is actually crucial for everyone to take a magnesium supplement. Unfortunately, oral magnesium is poorly absorbed. This is because of gastrointestinal disorders, medications, and the laxative effect of magnesium. Magnesium can be given intravenously, which will increase the levels by 100 percent.

Another very good way to bring up the magnesium level is to use magnesium oil. Magnesium oil (magnesium chloride) is a natural substance that can be applied to the skin or used in one's bath water, like Epsom salts.

Magnesium chloride is the first and most important item in any person's cancer treatment strategy. It takes about three to four months to drive up cellular magnesium levels, but within days patients will commonly experience its life-saving, healing effects.

Magnesium oil recommended by Dr. Mark Sircus is called "Ancient Minerals Magnesium Oil."http://www.canceriscurablenow.tv/newsletter/magnesium-part-your-anti-cancer-regime

❧ BETA GLUCAN

Beta-1,3-D glucan works by activating immune cells known as macrophages, neutrophiles, and natural killer cells. These cells are the immune system's first line of innate defense. They are responsible for finding, identifying, and consuming foreign substances in the body.

Bill Henderson recommends the Transfer Point brand of beta Glucan 1,3-D. Their glucan product is derived from the cell walls of baker's yeast, making it the precise substance for which the actual glucan macrophage receptor has been identified. The product is also very pure and of high quality, and they ship their product worldwide.

www.betterwayhealth.com

❧ SPIRULINA

Spirulina is a very powerful water plant with multiple benefits for the immune system. It provides an excellent source of carotenes, which are extremely beneficial for our immune system. They are imperative for the proper functioning of the immune system, helping correct defective DNA (which turns into cancer cells), and helping to correct bone marrow dysfunction.

It is the most powerful on this list of supplements and vitamins to boost the immune system because it reduces inflammation of the cells, which is known to turn healthy cells into cancer cells.

It helps correct autoimmune responses, stimulates all components of the immune system, and much more.

It also helps to protect against radiation damage (EMF) in our environment, which is a rapidly increasing problem for our immune systems.

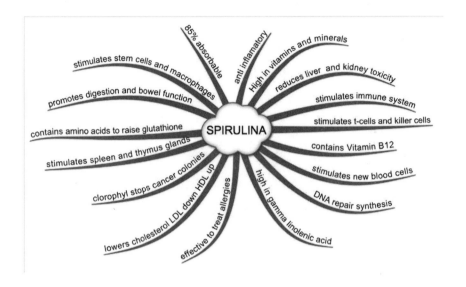

Exercise

☯ MASSAGE

Massage treatment is the manipulation of muscles and soft tissue through kneading, rubbing, pressing, etc.

Studies have shown that a massage will decrease stress, anxiety, depression, pain, and fatigue. Therefore, it is very beneficial in any cancer protocol. The connection among physical well-being, touch, and relaxation is very strong and can enhance the body's own abilities to heal.

Touch and close relationships are lacking in our society today, especially for elderly people. Massage can add tremendous benefits to every treatment protocol.

Special massages such as lymphatic drainage are successfully used in many cancer clinics to help the body move lymph through the lymphatic vessels, remove toxins, and boost the immune system.

There are some special situations with cancer patients that should always be considered before applying a massage treatment:Coagulation disorders, complicated by bruising and internal hemorrhage

- Low platelet count
- Medications: coumadin, acetylsalicylic acid. and heparin
- Metastases to bone, complicated by fracture
- Open wounds or radiation dermatitis can cause pain and infection

In these situations, avoiding massage or lightening the touch over regions of risk may prevent complications. No evidence suggests that massage therapy can spread cancer although avoiding direct pressure over a tumor is a sensible precaution.

Different massage techniques:

The Swedish massage consists of continuous systematic strokes, deep kneading, and stretching to loosen tight muscles and to reduce stress.

A deep tissue massage is applied with greater pressure and on deeper muscles than the classic Swedish massage. It generally focuses on a specific problem area.

Soft-tissue release is a technique that uses specific compression and precise extension, administered in a systematic manner, to release muscle spasms and scar tissue.

Neuromuscular therapy uses static pressure on specific myofascial points to relieve pain. This technique manipulates the soft tissue of the body (muscles, tendons, and connective tissue) and is thought to balance the central nervous system.

Lymphatic drainage is a very slow, light-touch, rhythmic massage that helps the body move lymph throughout the lymphatic vessels. It reduces edema and is also believed to remove toxins and boost the immunity.

Trigger-point therapy (myotherapy) consists of stretching the myofascial tissue through sustained, specific contact with pressure points which helps to release tension and pain.

Craniosacral therapy is a treatment approach that focuses on a gentle, hands-on technique used to evaluate and enhance the function of the cranial–sacral system. This hypothetical physiologic body system comprises the membranes and cerebrospinal fluid that surround and protect the brain and spinal cord. Craniosacral treatment is said to enhance the body's natural healing processes, improving the operation of the central nervous system, dissipating the negative effects of stress, enhancing health, and strengthening resistance to disease.

Shiatsu, meaning "finger pressure," is a Japanese massage—a form of physical manipulation of acupuncture points and meridians. The latter are thought to channel vital energy.

Acupressure is an ancient Asian healing art that uses the fingers on the surface of the skin to press key points that modulate energy flow through meridians and chakras. Manipulation of energy flow is speculated to stimulate the body's immune system and enhance self-healing.

Reflexology consists of firm pressure to specific points on the feet, hands, or ears. Reflexology is based on the principle that these regions contain links that correspond to every other part of the body.

☯ CARDIO

There are many benefits to exercise. The most important one for us to focus on is increased blood flow. When you exercise, your heart starts to pump more blood to the muscles that need it. This causes your pulse rate to increase, and you breathe more. This effect leads to higher oxygenation of the blood and better transportation of oxygen to all of the cells in the body. The same increased blood flow will then be able to carry all of the dead, weird, abnormal cells and other rubbish back to the liver for cleansing.

☯ LYMPHATIC

The lymphatic system drains the "waste" fluids from the cells. The word "lymph" comes from the Latin word "lympha," meaning water. Drinking fresh and clean water each day is mandatory to keep this system working. At least six to eight glasses of filtered water per day, in addition to any teas, are recommended.

The lymphatic system consists of glands in various parts of the body (such as the tonsils, the spleen, and the small glands in the armpits) linked by large lymph channels. The lymph glands' purpose is to filter out and destroy foreign substances and to produce antibodies and lymphatic cells for the lymph system. This system is the biggest tool your body has for maintaining its immunity to disease.

The blood stream uses the heart to pump blood around the body. So, because there is no "heart" to pump the lymphatic system, how does it work?

MUSCLE MOVEMENT!

The flow of the lymphatic fluids is regulated by valves, but it is generated through the system by BODY MOVEMENT. That is why it is so important to KEEP MOVING. Any form of exercise is better than none. Surprisingly, simply walking is almost as good as running and going to the gym, in this respect.

Regular physical activity, performed nearly every day of the week, reduces the risk of developing or dying from some form of degenerative disease.

- Reduces the risk of heart disease
- Reduces the risk of developing diabetes
- Reduces the risk of high blood pressure
- Reduces the risk of developing cancer
- Reduces the feelings of anxiety and depression
- Promotes recovery and physical well-being

Exercise is a mandatory treatment for every cancer patient. Unfortunately, many cancer patients are so weak that daily exercise is very difficult to perform. Dr. Finn Scott Anderson from the Hummlegaarden clinic in Denmark says in the movie that exercise is chemotherapy for your cancer.

So, depending on the strength of the patient, exercise should be a part of the patient's daily routine. Just a 10-minute walk is very beneficial, and the combination of walking barefoot in the sunlight will increase the benefits immensely.

Once the patient improves, walking, swimming, cycling, and dancing are wonderful exercise regimens.

Yoga and stretching are also very beneficial and can be performed at many different levels of fitness.

☯ LYMPHATIC EXERCISE

A mini trampoline is a very effective tool. Rebounding on a mini trampoline benefits lymphatic circulation by stimulating the millions of one-way valves in the lymphatic system. Through the gravitational pull, toxins get squeezed out of the estimated 60 trillion cells in our bodies. The short weightlessness in the air promotes the movements of nutrients into the cells. This whole process is like exercising every cell in the body.

The lymphatic system is the rubbish bin of the body. Lymphatic vessels are located all over the body but they are more concentrated in certain areas, such as the breasts. Therefore, women should obtain a mini trampoline and conduct daily rebounding sessions, especially if they have breast cancer.

NASA says rebounding is as much as 68 percent more efficient than jogging on a treadmill. Therefore, rebounding only three to five minutes, twice a day, will advance both men and women from a category 1 fitness level to a category 2 or 3, as long as one of those minutes consists of aerobic bouncing as vigorously as possible.

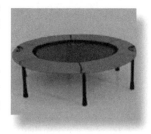

This enhances the body's immune capacity for fighting any current disease, destroying cancer cells, eliminating antigens, and preventing future illness.

Participating in a support group will also help you stay focused and achieve your goals.

Exercise needs to be determined on an individual basis, according to strength and physical conditions. Never overdo it as this would cost the already burdened body too much energy.

☯ YOGA

There are three main structures of yoga: yoga exercise, breathing, and meditation. The ancient yogis believed in being in harmony with oneself and the environment through the integration of body, mind, and spirit; this helped them achieve and maintain balance in their life.

There is a strong mind and body connection which, when harmonized, can result in mental and physical benefits.

Areas where different yoga exercises or asana are extremely effective:

- Increasing overall flexibilityIncreasing lubrication of joints, ligaments, and tendonsMassaging all organs of the body—yoga is the only activity that massages all of the internal glands and organs of the body.

- Complete detoxification—the stretching of muscles and joints and the massaging of the internal organ ensures optimal blood supply to all cells. This helps to flush out toxins.

- Excellent toning of the musclesHelps to release stressMakes the body-mind connectionYoga can be easily practiced at home or at one of the many yoga centers around the world.

Oxygenation

☯ BREATHING

Oxygen is what keeps your body alive. Every cell in your body needs oxygen to produce energy. A few minutes without oxygen will not only cause cells to die, but eventually the entire body will die.

On the contrary, cancer cells require a lot less oxygen for their metabolism to produce energy. As determined by Dr. Otto Warburg, they are able to derive their energy through a fermentation process of blood sugar; therefore, any oxygen-deprived cells can revert to their "primitive" state.

Therefore, it is only logical that a body saturated with oxygen functions so much better and is capable of aiding in the elimination of cancer cell production.

There are many ways to increase the cellular oxygen level.

☯ WALKING / HUMMING

The first method is also the cheapest, **exercise**. Humming while you walk increases the oxygen intake manifold. The vibrations from humming sooth the nerves while helping to increase the flow of oxygen through the body.

We must also learn to breathe properly. Most people breathe very shallowly. According to the University of Missouri-Kansas City, oxygen levels can also drop 20 percent as we age, partially due to poor breathing habits.

Most of the yoga centers teach highly valuable breathings techniques. The problem is you must form a habit by practicing these techniques on a daily basis.

HYPERBARIC OXYGEN

Different oxygenating therapies saturate the body with oxygen, such as hyperbaric oxygen therapy, ozone therapy, and hydrogen peroxide therapy. The total amount of available oxygen in the blood is also increased through the use of gas, sometimes at high pressures (HPOT Hyperbaric Chamber).

Benefits of Hyperbaric Oxygen Treatment:

This treatment boosts the immune system response through the functionality of white blood cells.

White blood cell function is based upon the use of oxygen. Through the boost of high oxygen, the ability to cause cytotoxicity (killing off) of abnormal cells and intruders (bacteria, viruses) is increased. Infections are always present in patients with cancer.

Oxygen, in the presence of a therapeutic dose of vitamin C, generates hydrogen peroxide radical. This radical cannot be neutralized by catalase (enzyme), which is not readily available in solid tumors. This, in turn, causes direct poisoning of the cancer cell metabolism and results in cancer cell destruction.

Hyperbaric oxygen can potentiate the effectiveness of chemotherapy, sensitizing the tumor cells to be more vulnerable.

Hyperbaric oxygen can also reduce inflammation and edema caused by the tumor. In the situation of tumor death, it reduces the inflammatory response to tumor necrosis and the complications associated with the death of the tumor cell.

Hyperbaric oxygen can also reduce other localized inflammatory responses to treatment.

In compromised tissues, HBOT can stimulate angiogenesis and facilitate the healing of tissues that have undergone surgery or have been damaged as a result of therapy.

It also greatly increases oxygen concentration in all body tissues (up to 25 times). Red blood cells are carriers of oxygen, and not only are they saturated, but also the serum is itself is saturated, facilitating the delivery of oxygen to areas that cannot be reached by the red blood cells.

There is a rebound arterial dilation after HBOT, resulting in an increased blood vessel diameter greater than when therapy began, which improves blood flow to compromised tissues.

This treatment increases (by 8 times) the body's natural production of STEM cells, which are called into action from the bone marrow to repair organs and tissues and generate new components for the production of red blood cells, white blood cells, and platelets.

This treatment provides an abundant amount of oxygen for the liver and individual cellular detoxification mechanisms, which are oxygen-dependent during the internal cleansing process.

You can obtain information about a hyperbaric center near you by phone or e-mail at the International Hyperbaric Association, Inc. website.

http://www.ihausa.org

☯ ARDENNE

Dr. Manfred von Ardenne is the founder of the Oxygen Multi-Step Therapy. He described a unique protocol, involving the delivery of oxygen at the rate of six to eight liters per minute for a full two-hour period and repeated daily for 18 consecutive days. It is a very simple method and can be done at home by using oxygen with a face mask and breathing bag.

Dr. Ardenne was a student of Dr. Otto Warburg, who received the 1931 Nobel Prize for proving that cancer is anaerobic; it cannot survive in a high-oxygen environment.

Most diseases, whether resulting from an allergy, infection, or toxicity, cause edema, or the swelling of the smallest blood vessels.

This swelling reduces blood flow as well as the rate at which oxygen is dissolved in the blood stream and can reach the tissues. As the reduction in tissue oxygenation continues, all body functions are compromised.

☯ HYDROGEN PEROXIDE

Hydrogen peroxide has the chemical formula of H_2O_2 and contains one more atom of oxygen than water (H_2O).

When ozone mixes with moisture in the air, it forms hydrogen peroxide, which comes down in rain and snow. It occurs naturally in fresh fruits and vegetables—some of it comes from rain and some is manufactured during photosynthesis. Hydrogen peroxide is also found in mother's milk, with an especially high concentration in colostrum (the first milk secreted right after birth).

We all have probably witnessed the bubbling of hydrogen peroxide when it comes in contact with a bacteria-laden cut or even our toothbrush we want to clean. The bubbles are the oxygen that is released and the bacteria being killed.

Lactobacillus, which is found in our colon, produces hydrogen peroxide to destroy harmful bacteria and viruses.

When hydrogen peroxide comes in contact with other substances, it splits readily into oxygen and water. This oxygen atom is then very reactive and referred to as a free radical. Our body creates and uses free radicals to kill harmful bacteria, viruses, and fungi. The same reaction happens with the free oxygen from the hydrogen peroxide—it kills unwanted intruders.

It is proven that the spread of cancer cells is inversely proportional to the amount of oxygen around the cancer cells. If cancer cells get enough oxygen, they die.

It is thought that hydrogen peroxide kills cancer cells because cancer cells do not have the mechanism to break down hydrogen peroxide that healthy cells have.

Hydrogen peroxide is used either orally or intravenously. One possible way in which intravenous hydrogen peroxide can treat cancer is by releasing pure oxygen in the body. By saturating the cells and tissues with oxygen, hydrogen peroxide promotes healthy, oxygen-based metabolism.

Hydrogen peroxide therapy needs to be administered by a physician.

There are now numerous hydrogen peroxide products on the market. Some are simply peroxide that has been flavored and mixed with sea minerals, aloe vera, inner tree bark, or other ingredients to make the peroxide more palatable (Superoxy, Oxy Toddy, etc.).

http://www.superoxy.com

http://www.eagle-min.com/oxtod.htm

☯ OZONE

What is ozone therapy?

Ozone is a molecule with three atoms of oxygen attached together, or O3. The oxygen molecule you are breathing right now is made up of two atoms of oxygen attached together, or O2. They seem similar; however, they have completely different effects on the human body.

Many believe it to be the most promising, safe, and generally efficacious treatment for major degenerative diseases, from AIDS and chronic fatigue to cancer and arthritis.

Medical ozone differs from atmospheric ozone in that it is pure and concentrated. Atmospheric ozone is combined with nitrous oxide and sulfur oxide and is, therefore, dangerous.

Ozone therapy is widely practiced in Europe, but there are some doctors who offer ozone therapy in the United States.

Go to this website for a list of physicians:
http://www.oxygenhealingtherapies.com

Benefits of ozone therapy:

- Activation of white blood cells to kill bacteria
- Oxygenation of the cells and tissues
- Increase in mitochondrial ATP production
- Improves enzyme processes
- Kills unwanted bacteria
- Improves circulation through blood thinning

"First of all, it stimulates the production of white blood cells and increases the production of interferon, interleuken-2, and tumor necrosis factor, which the body uses to fight infections and cancer. It is anti-neoplastic, which means that it inhibits the growth of tumors. One study performed at Baylor University in Texas, in 1962, determined that ozone can help to kill tumors and enhance the effect of different types of anti-tumor drugs. Ozone kills bacteria and viruses. In addition, it increases the amount of oxygen in the blood and helps deliver oxygen to all of the cells in the body. It also helps degrade petrochemicals. This includes different toxins that one might have in the body due to the environment or food eaten. It helps dissolve and eliminate them from the body; hence, it lightens the body's toxic load. It also increases red blood cell membrane distensability, making it more flexible. This is one way it is used in the treatment of heart disease. ...

How is ozone therapy administered?

An ozone mixture is introduced into a fixed volume of the patient's blood outside of the body and then promptly re-infused into the patient. This method, mainly used in Germany, is called autohemotherapy.

Another common method is to administer ozone rectally, which is called ozone insufflation. A catheter is put into the colon and gas from an ozone machine is allowed in at a determined concentration and flow rate. After oxygen-ozone mixtures are absorbed through the wall of the large intestine, they enter the bloodstream and result in a PaO2 increase within the entire body, raising PaO2 almost 100 percent higher than oxygen alone would, and there are no adverse effects.

The oxygen-ozone mixtures are absorbed through the large intestine into the bloodstream. Since 1936, there have been positive effects on diseases of the colon and rectum noted. The ozone renews the mucous lining and gets to the bacterial infestation that has infiltrated the tissues of the colon.

Other methods of ozone treatments are direct intra-arterial and intravenous application, vaginal insufflation / urethral insufflation, ear insufflation, intramuscular injection, body ozone exposure in a sauna, and different topical applications.

Detoxification

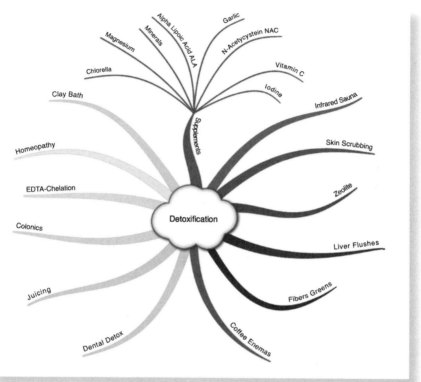

Detoxification is a very important factor in dealing with disease in general but especially cancer.

Nowadays, every person has a body overloaded with toxins. According to the EWG, babies are already born with more than 250 toxins in their umbilical cord.

Detoxification is mandatory for everyone. Depending on the toxins and the physical condition of the patient, there are several ways to detoxify the body.

An optimal detoxification program should consider these points:

- Identify and get rid of toxins
- Fix your gut—a source of high toxicity for many

- Get moving—to help your blood and lymphatic circulation do its job
- Get your liver and detox system working
- Eat a healthy organic diet without any allergens
- Drink plenty of fresh, toxin-free water
- Avoid stimulants like coffee, alcohol, drugs, and nicotine
- Detox your mind, heart, and spirit

With every kind of detoxification program, when the toxins are released, the patient can experience side effects like headache, dizziness, nausea, stomach ache, etc. If you have any problems, please contact a physician for assistance. Immediately reduce the amount you are taking as the released toxin load is also a burden on the body. Your elimination system also needs to be fully functional; otherwise, the toxins just get flushed out of the liver to get stuck in the intestines. Therefore, a diet high in fiber and good quality water is very important to successfully eliminate the toxins. In many cases, it is also necessary to support the liver and kidneys as they are often stressed during a detoxification process. Please consult your physician!

Certain supplements are also needed to combine with any of the detoxification methods listed below:

Glutathione (GSH) is the body's most important and prevalent antioxidant. It plays a critical role in neutralizing harmful free radicals, protecting the body from toxic substances and removing mercury.

It takes two molecules of glutathione to escort one atom of mercury out of the body. This action results in a net loss of the body's most powerful and critically important antioxidant!

As mentioned earlier, oral glutathione will not increasing the level of it in the body. However, N-acetyl cysteine, spirulina, and whey protein will increase glutathione levels.

N-acetyl cysteine (NAC) plays a vital role in supporting the body's ability to remove mercury. It increases the body's natural level of glutathione, which is the most important mercury removing antioxidant. NAC is also a powerful antioxidant by itself.

Alpha lipoic acid (ALA) is the most biologically active form of lipoic acid and is the form that the body produces naturally. ALA is a powerful antioxidant and mercury chelator. It is fat-soluble, crosses the blood/brain barrier, and chelates mercury in the central nervous system.

Minerals are very important to support any detoxification process. First, they are flushed out from the body through the heavy metals, and, second, they are also flushed out through the detoxification process. They need to be replenished daily as they are water-soluble; therefore, they are not effectively stored in the body.

Magnesium is a crucial factor in the natural self-cleansing and detoxification response of the body. Magnesium is not a chelator itself, but it is necessary for detoxing and chelation.

Chlorella traps toxic metals in the GI tract, performs a cleansing action on the bowel and other elimination channels, protects the liver, and keeps the blood clean.

Vitamin C

Garlic

Iodine promotes the excretion of all heavy metals, including aluminum and the halides, bromide, and fluoride. Seek professional advice before supplementing iodine, and get your iodine levels tested.

The list of detoxification methods is not complete but will hopefully be a helpful start.

☯ ENEMAS

Enemas are "fluids injected into the rectum for the purpose of clearing out the bowel or for administering drugs or food."

The enema is one of the oldest medical procedures still in use today. The use of coffee enemas began at least as early as 1917 and was found in the prestigious Merck Manual until 1972.

When a coffee enema is used, the caffeine in the coffee is absorbed into the system. It then travels directly to the liver where it becomes a very strong detoxicant. Because the enema is generally held for 15 minutes and all of the blood in the body passes through the liver every three minutes, "these enemas represent a form of dialysis of blood across the gut wall."

What you need:

- A stainless steel enema bucket (colonic kit)
- Organic, caffeinated coffee
- Uncontaminated, filtered water
- Organic, non-bleached coffee filters

Procedure:

- Cook 0.5 L of a normal, strong coffee in a pot for 10 minutes.
- Let the coffee cool to a lukewarm temperature. Be careful not to use the coffee while it is still hot or after it becomes too cold. It should be very close to normal body temperature, which is 36.8C.
- Fill your enema kit with the coffee, but make sure that you do not have any coffee grounds in your liquid.
- Prepare a place in the bathroom where you can lay on a towel.
- Follow the instructions of your enema kit. Lie on your right side and gently insert the tip very slowly.
- Allow the coffee to flow in.
- Retain the enema for 15 minutes, changing sides after 5 minutes.
- Pass the time by reading a book or meditating; do not attempt to walk around the house.
- Release the contents into the toilet after 15 minutes or so.
- Do not forget to wash the enema kit thoroughly with soap and water after every use.
- This procedure is easier if you perform the enema after a bowel movement. At first, you may have difficulties holding the coffee in for 15 minutes but don't get discouraged.

- Be patient—practice makes perfect.

How often should you do a coffee enema?

According to the Gerson Therapy, coffee enemas are done at least three times per day and up to as many as six times. This is a lot for many patients. Many doctors recommend one enema per day for a prolonged period of time, which can be months or years.

Never forget to replenish your mineral status after enema treatments.

☯ CLAY

Bentonite clay, referred to as "healing clay," is a safe, effective, and natural method of detoxification. It binds heavy metals, radiation, chemicals, pathogens, and many other toxins. Clay has powerful drawing and absorptive capabilities.

The skin is the largest eliminative organ of the human body.

Detoxification bath:

The minerals in clay that are mostly negatively charged literally draw the positively charged heavy metals to it and eliminate them through the skin. Immersing oneself fully in a warm clay bath relaxes muscles and opens the pores of the skin, allowing the clay to absorb impurities and unhealthy pollutants.

Taking a clay bath twice a week has a dramatic effect in reducing heavy metals. Clay baths add no stress to the liver and are very easy to do in the comfort of your own home. The bath should be as hot as possible.

Dissolve one to twelve cups of clay in the bath and soak in it for 15 to 30 minutes. Drinking edible clay 30 minutes before the bath supports the detoxification process.

Never forget to replenish your mineral status after clay treatments.

Edible clay can be used orally:

Through the micron small particles of the clay, it is possible for the edible clay to permeate the blood stream and pull out toxins.

The following benefits are achieved:

- Detoxification of the digestive system (The absorptive action of clay pulls contaminants from the body.)
- Reduction in bacterial, organic, and non-organic toxicity
- Elimination of internal parasites (digestive tracts)
- Immune system support (Clay used internally stimulates the body's elimination system and supports organ function.)
- Fixes free oxygen in the blood stream (occurs once the liver has been restored to full function)
- Increases T-cell count
- Fights free radicals
- Liver detoxification
- Treats stomach aches and bacterial food poisoning
- Acts as an alkalizing agent in the body

The recommended dose is around one teaspoon in the morning on an empty stomach.

Please be aware:

If you are currently under chemotherapy or radiation, calcium montmorillonite clay will likely conflict with your treatment in its effort to pull poisons out of the body. However, this high quality clay is often used AFTER these types of treatments—but you should always consult your doctor first. Chemotherapy is a heavy metal—platinum. Calcium montmorillonite clay may remove this quite effectively, along with other metals that do not belong in the body.

☯ ZEOLITE

Zeolites are natural volcanic minerals with a unique, complex crystalline structure. Zeolite's honey comb framework of cavities and channels (like cages) works at the cellular level, trapping heavy metals and toxins. In fact, because it is one of the few negatively charged minerals in nature, zeolites act as magnets, drawing positively charged toxins to it, capturing them in its cage, and removing them from the body.

As the zeolite moves through the body, the negative charge within its pores becomes neutralized while it attracts and captures the positively charged heavy metal ions. Once these toxins are trapped, they stay locked within the zeolite and are passed safely out of the body.

The end result of using zeolite is that it improves the efficiency of our bodies' toxin defense systems by trapping and removing harmful metals and toxins and supporting the body's natural detoxification processes.

Those effects initially can include detoxification and/or healing changes. Some may get a return of old symptoms as the body starts to deal with the accumulated toxins from years of living. This can lead to significantly increased frequency of urination, bowel movements, skin rashes, or even headaches in some, which is related to the dose taken. Consequently, many are advised to start out with lower doses initially to limit the detoxification symptoms.

Zeolite is not totally selective to heavy metals and binds essential minerals in small amounts too. It is necessary to take a mineral supplement while on zeolite detoxification.

☯ JUICES

All medical authorities acknowledge the benefits of consuming fresh, green juices.

Green foods contain chlorophyll, which very closely resembles hemoglobin. (Hemoglobin carries oxygen in our blood.) Some research is now suggesting that chlorophyll can be converted to hemoglobin, and may increase the flow of oxygen to all parts of the body.

An oxygen-rich milieu is very important because it is detrimental to the fight against bad bacteria and cancer cells.

Green foods are very high in trace minerals. They are also rich in essential amino acids, which act as building blocks for the immune system. Importantly, they are rich in phtyonutrients, which are capable of initiating chemical reactions. These enzymes initiate cleansing, detoxifying, and rebuilding the body, while enhancing the immune system.

As previously mentioned in the chapter on diet, green foods are very alkaline and will normalize the body to a healthy pH of more than seven.

❂ CHELATION

Chelation is a chemical process in which a metal or mineral such as lead, mercury, or calcium is bonded to another substance. For this process, a weak acid EDTA is used. EDTA is a synthetic amino acid and is often used as a food preservative.

In chelation therapy, EDTA can be used orally or intravenously.

EDTA therapy is approved by the FDA for removing heavy lead poisoning.

"Every human being today would live longer, be more intelligent, have a higher level of health, and respond better to any remedy if they chose to follow an EDTA chelation therapy program," says Dr. Garry Gordon, who is one of the presenters in our movie.

Contact a physician who offers this type of program to participate in chelation therapy.

If you would like to read more about chelation therapy, there is a wonderful book available by David Jay Brown and Garry Gordon,

MD, called *Detox with Oral Chelation: Protecting Yourself from Lead, Mercury, & Other Environmental Toxins*.

☯ CHLORELLA

Chlorella is a fresh water, single-celled, green algae. It contains vitamins, minerals, amino acids, and chlorophyll, to name its most important components. Chlorella helps the body to detoxify. It is found that the rough, fibrous material in the outer shell binds the toxins and carries them out of the body.

As chlorella also contains more than 12 percent chlorophyll, it rapidly increases the oxygenation of the blood.

How much chlorella should you take?

For general maintenance, 3 to 5 grams per day is adequate. Fighting cancer requires around 20 grams per day.

As with every detoxification program, side effects can occur. The detox reactions come from the release of more toxins than the chlorella can bind. Therefore decreasing the dose can reduce the side effects.

☯ VITAMIN C

Vitamin C is an essential nutrient of the body. Our body does not synthesize vitamin C like rats and mice do; therefore, it needs to be taken in through our daily food or by supplementation.

Vitamin C, or ascorbic acid, is a powerful antioxidant and demonstrates the ability to neutralize a wide variety of toxic substances. As many toxins have been shown to have cancer-causing effects, it is necessary to take additional vitamin C in the form of a supplement.

When taken in high doses, vitamin C can easily upset one's digestive system and cause diarrhea and stomach pain. To eliminate this problem, it is important to take vitamin C in its buffered form.

The recommended daily allowance of vitamin C is totally outdated. Studies indicate that a starting dose should be a minimum of 2,000 mg per day or more.

Dr. Garry Gordon and Dr. Conneally recommend a vitamin C supplement which can be taken orally in very high doses without any kind of stomach problems.

One of the most valuable books on the market on vitamin C is *Curing the Incurable: Vitamin C, Infectious Diseases, and Toxins* by Thomas Levy, MD, JD. LINK

High doses of intravenous vitamin C were common practice in many clinics we visited—all with a high success rate in treating cancer.

☯ GARLIC

Garlic is a powerful, yet natural, detoxifier. Garlic contains numerous sulphur components, including the most valuable sulph-hydryl groups, which oxidize mercury, cadmium, and lead, making them water-soluble. Once these metals are water-soluble, it is easy for the body to eliminate them.

Garlic also contains alliin, which is transformed into allicin, a potent antimicrobial agent.

Selenium is an ingredient in garlic that protects the body from mercury toxicity.

For centuries, garlic has been a very valuable, natural remedy and should not be forgotten in any health protocol.

☯ LIVER FLUSHES

A liver flush or liver cleanse is interchangeable with a gallbladder cleanse. The goal is to remove small, uncalcified gallstones that remain undetected by diagnostic testing. The liver flush can also help to treat allergies, high cholesterol, malnutrition, and cancer.

A typical liver cleanse involves consuming a large quantity of fruit juice followed by a special concoction that flushes the liver and gallbladder of accumulated toxins. This concoction mostly consists of olive oil, Epsom salts, and lemon juice.

The liver cleanse is normally done over a two-day period and can be done from home. (You don't want to leave the house.) People who are known to have stones should not attempt the gallbladder or liver flush because of the risk of obstruction. The presence of abdominal pain, nausea, or vomiting is absolutely contraindications for liver cleanse and liver-gallbladder flush.

Liver flushes are very beneficial in eliminating toxins from the liver and gallbladder. However, you should definitely consult your doctor before doing a liver/gallbladder flush.

☯ COLONICS

Colonics is a therapy where the entire length of the colon is flushed with water. Colonics are done by a trained colon hydrotherapist and require professional equipment. Colonics can get rid of toxic waste build up. It is an excellent method of eliminating toxins and improving digestion, sleep patterns, energy levels, and skin conditions.

Colonics are a quick way to clean out the colon; however, colonics should not been done too often and are not remedies for ongoing detoxification.

☯ SKIN SCRUBBING

Hydrotherapy is detoxification via the skin through body brushing.

Gently brush your skin with a dry loofah sponge. This massage increases the circulation of blood and lymph and aids in the detox process. Using gentle strokes and beginning with the soles of your feet, move up your legs, hips, and abdomen, then continue with your arms from fingertips to shoulders, across your torso and back, finally finishing with your neck. Follow with a nice shower or a bath of your choice.

Bathing in Dr. Gordon's "Beyond Clean" Epsom salts and magnesium bath has a very detoxifying result, especially for radiation.

> *The doctor of the future will give no medicine, but will interest his patients in the care of the human frame, in diet and the cause and prevention of disease.*
>
> *-Thomas Edison*

☯ FIBERS / GREENS

Fibers are the portion of a plant that our bodies cannot digest or absorb. Nevertheless, fiber has an essential purpose in our diet.

There are two types of fibers available:

- Soluble fiber, which dissolves in water to form a gel-like material. It is found in oats, peas, beans, apples, citrus fruits, carrots, barley, and psyllium.
- Insoluble fiber promotes the movement of material through the digestive tract. It increases stool bulk and aids in alleviating constipation. It is found in brown rice, whole grains, bran, nuts, and many vegetables.

Benefits of fiber in our diet:

- Eliminates toxins with an easy and fast passage through the intestinal tractRegulates blood sugar by trapping carbohydrates and slowing absorption of glucoseLowers total and LDL cholesterolSimulates intestinal fermentation production of short-chain fatty acids, which may reduce the risk of colorectal cancer

☯ HOMEOPATHIC

Many complex homeopathic remedies are used for detoxification.

The most widely used supplement we came across is the "Detox Kit" by HEEL. It consists of three bottles; each one addresses a different detoxification function of the body.

- Lymphomysot helps maintain blood circulation to the peripheral areas of the body (legs, hands, and feet), assists or aids in the treatment of fluid retention, and helps with the detoxification process.
- Nux vomica-Homaccord is a liver tonic. It aids in digestion and also assists in detoxification.
- Reneel is a kidney tonic and helps to maintain proper kidney function. It also assists in detoxification.

It is obvious that this product uses three different substances to support the three main detoxifying organs: the lymph system, liver, and kidneys.

Benefits:

- A complete detoxification program for all states of toxic overloadStimulates the body's natural drainage process to allow auto-regulation and elimination of toxinsCan be used singularly or in any combination, depending on the symptomsContains medicines of elimination and drainage for the liver, kidneys, and lymphatic systemA treatment for rapid detoxification of chemicals, drugs, and medicationMay be suitable for long-term treatment in chronic diseasesWill help reduce the toxicity symptoms of chemotherapy

☯ INFRARED SAUNA

Most of the clinics we visited use infrared sauna to detoxify their patients' bodies.

Sweating is the body's safe and natural way to flush out toxins. Research has long since proven that toxic substances, including heavy metals, are secreted from the body through sweat. Therefore, the more one can safely sweat (while maintaining proper hydration), the more toxins will be released from the body. In a sauna detox, sweat carries toxins out of the body through the pores.

Every sauna that induces sweating will detoxify. The benefits of an infrared sauna involve the amount of toxins that are released—around 20 percent compared to 4 percent of a normal sauna. The infrared sauna not only heats up the outer layers of skin but also goes far deeper into the tissues and stimulates the immune system too.

In the infrared sauna, 80 to 85 percent of the sweat is water, with the non-water portion being principally cholesterol, fat-soluble toxins, toxic heavy metals, sulfuric acid, sodium, ammonia, and uric acid. Using the skin as an essential aspect of chelation therapy is important and makes absolute perfect sense.

According to Dr. Robert O. Young, the infrared sauna provides the following benefits:

> Speeds up metabolic processes of vital organs and glands, including endocrine glandsInhibits the development of fungi, yeasts, bacteria, and molds and creates a fever reaction of rising temperature that neutralizes themIncreases the number of leukocytes in the bloodPlaces a demand on the heart to work harder, thus exercising it and also producing a drop in diastolic blood pressure (the low side)Stimulates dilation of peripheral blood vessels, relieving pain (including muscle pain) and speeding the healing of sprains, arthritis, and peripheral vascular disease symptomsPromotes relaxation thereby creating a feeling of well-being Daily sauna is recommended if the physical condition of the patient will tolerate it.

An infrared sauna is not a cheap investment but definitely one that is worthwhile because it can be used by the whole family and all of your friends.

http://www.canceriscurablenow.tv/newsletter/no-emf-far-inrared-sauna-new-breakthrough

☯ DENTAL DETOX

Amalgam fillings, which are made of mercury, add tremendously to your overall toxic load. Day by day, mercury is leaking out of these fillings and poisoning your system.

Mercury fillings have been proven to be neurotoxic, embryotoxic, mutagenic, and immunotoxic. In simple terms, mercury weakens the immune system, has adverse effects on the function of the central and peripheral nervous system, has toxic effects on the embryo, and increases the frequency of mutation.

There is no healing possible without removing the constant poisoning of the system through mercury fillings.

Safe removal of these fillings is very often the only solution to minimize the toxic load of the body. But be careful because taking out the amalgam needs to be done by a professional who knows what they are dealing with—A HIGHLY TOXIC SUBSTANCE!

We recommend a biological dentist who takes precautionary measures in removing amalgam fillings. It is very beneficial if the dentist has a special, built-in air filter system to minimize the inhalation of mercury. Some dentists even administer IV vitamin C during this procedure to detox the body and keep the toxic exposure at a minimum.

Another factor that needs to be addressed in your mouth is chronic inflammation known as gum disease. Chronic inflammation is responsible for many chronic diseases, including cancer.

Gum disease includes gingivitis and periodontitis.

Gingivitis is the inflammation of the gum caused by bacterial build up. The gum gets swollen, red, and bleeds easily. Good oral hygiene and proper diet can eliminate this problem.

Periodontitis is much more serious because the plaque which used to be around the tooth has now spread below the gum line. Toxins produced by the bacteria trigger chronic inflammation and are a heavy burden to the immune system. In addition, heart disease, diabetes, and respiratory disease are associated with periodontitis.

> *Dr. Dominique Michaud of the Harvard School of Public Health in Boston said, "Men with a history of periodontal disease had a 64 percent increased risk of pancreatic cancer than men with no history."*

If you have problems with bleeding gums, please see a biological dentist.

Alkaline

All functions of the body are very well balanced, so even the slightest deviation away from the normal range will cause havoc within the whole system. One of these systems is our pH, which is measured on a scale from 1 to 14, where 1 is very acidic and 14 is very alkaline; midway (7) would be neutral. Our normal blood pH is about 7.4, which is slightly alkaline.

Our body's pH controls the activity of every metabolic function occurring within our body. Our pH is active within the body's electrical system and intracellular activity and is the way our body utilizes enzymes, minerals, and vitamins. Cancer cells have a lower pH than surrounding tissues.

Through our diet of high sugar and processed food, the pH of most people is very acidic. Everyone can test a urine sample with pH test strips.

Unfortunately, our cells need this strictly balanced pH system to work properly. In an acidic environment, it is like they are paralyzed and can't fulfill their normal duty.

The following are some methods for changing the body's pH.

☯ SODIUM BICARBONATE

Sodium bicarbonate, also known as baking soda, has an alkaline pH. It is a natural antacid and a cheap, but very effective, way of balancing the pH.

Oral $NaHCO_3$ selectively increased the pH of tumors and reduced the formation of spontaneous metastases of breast cancer in experimental mice. $NaHCO_3$ therapy also reduced the rate of lymph node involvement and significantly reduced the formation of hepatic metastases.

At the University of Arizona, Robert J. Gillies and his colleagues have demonstrated that sodium bicarbonate increases tumor pH (i.e., makes it more alkaline) and also inhibits spontaneous metastases (Robey 2009). They showed that oral sodium bicarbonate increased the pH of tumors and also reduced the formation of spontaneous metastases in mice with breast cancer. It also reduced the rate of lymph node involvement.

At a pH slightly above 7.4, cancer cells become dormant and at a pH level of 8.5, cancer cells will die while healthy cells will live. This has given rise to a variety of treatments based on increasing the alkalinity of the tissues, such as a vegetarian diet, the drinking of fresh fruit and vegetable juices, and dietary supplementation with alkaline minerals such as calcium, potassium, magnesium, cesium, and rubidium. But nothing can compare to the instant alkalizing power of sodium bicarbonate for safe and effective treatment of cancer.

High quality baking soda from the health food store is mixed with water and taken on an empty stomach. Most of the time, after a few days, a balanced pH is achieved.

Sodium bicarbonate should never be considered as a standalone treatment. It should be used in conjunction with a full protocol.

Dr. Simoncini, an oncologist in Rome, Italy, has pioneered sodium bicarbonate ($NaHCO_3$) therapy as a means to treat cancer.

The theory behind his treatment is that the formation and spreading of tumors is simply the result of the presence of a fungus.

The basic concept is the administration of a solution with a high content of sodium bicarbonate directly into the tumors. These are susceptible to regression only if one destroys the fungal colonies.

If it is not possible to get the injection directly into the tumor, Dr. Simoncini places a small catheter directly into the artery that nourishes the tumor and administers high doses of sodium bicarbonate to the deepest recesses of the tumor.

Sodium bicarbonate, unlike other anti-fungal remedies to which the fungus can become immune, is extremely diffusible and retains its ability to penetrate the tumor because of the speed at which the sodium bicarbonate disintegrates the tumor. This speed makes fungi's adaptability impossible, rendering it defenseless.

Dr.Simoncini says that almost all organs can be treated and can benefit from bicarbonate salts therapy, which is harmless, fast and effective—with the exception of some bone areas such as vertebrae and ribs, where the scarce arterial irrigation does not allow sufficient dosage to reach the targets.

Dr.Simoncini wrote the book *Cancer is a Fungus: A Revolution in Tumor Therapy*, which can be ordered via his website:

www.cancerisafugus.com

☯ DIET / JUICING / GREENS

The best way to change your pH is through diet.

A basic rule to achieve and maintain a pH balance is to eat 80 percent alkaline- and 20 percent acid-forming foods and drinks each day.

LIST OF ALKALIZING FOODS:

Alkalizing Vegetables
Alfalfa, barley grass, beet greens, beets, broccoli, cabbage, carrots, cauliflower, celery, chard, chlorella, cucumbers, dandelions, dulce, eggplant, fermented veggies, garlic, green beans, kale, kohlrabi, lettuce, mushrooms, mustard greens, onions, parsnip, peas, peppers, pumpkin, radishes, sea veggies, spinach, spirulina, sprouts, sweet potatoes, watercress, tomatoes, wheat grass, and wild greens**Alkalizing Protein**
Almonds, chestnuts, millet, tempeh, and whey protein powder

Alkalizing Fruits
Apples, apricots, avocados, bananas, berries, cherries, fresh coconut, currants, dried dates, dried figs, grapes, grapefruit,

honeydew melon, lemons, limes, tangerines, tropical fruits, and watermelon

Other Alkalizing Food Products
Alkaline water, apple cider vinegar, bee pollen, green juices, probiotic cultures, veggie juices, and soured dairy products

LIST OF ACIDIFYING FOODS:

Acidifying Vegetables
Corn, lentils, olives, and winter squash

Acidifying Fruits
Cranberries and canned fruits

Acidifying Grains and Grain Products
Amaranth, barley, oat bran, wheat bran, bread, corn, cornstarch, flour, hemp seed flour, kamut, noodles, pasta, oatmeal, rolled oats, all rice, rice cakes, rye, spelt, wheat germ, and wheat

Acidifying Beans and Legumes
Almond milk, black beans, chick peas, green peas, kidney beans, lentils, pinto beans, red beans, rice milk, soybeans, soy milk, and white beans**Acidifying Dairy**
Butter, cheese, ice cream, and ice milk

Acidifying Nuts and Butters
Cashews, peanut butter, peanuts, pecans, tahini, and walnuts

Acidifying Animal Protein
Bacon, beef, carp, clams, cod, fish, lamb, lobster, mussels, oyster, pork, rabbit, salmon, sausage, scallops, shellfish, shrimp, tuna, turkey, veal, and venison

Acidifying Fats and Oils
Avocado oil, butter, canola oil, corn oil, flax oil, hemp seed oil, lard, olive oil, safflower oil, sesame oil, and sunflower oil

Acidifying Sweeteners
Sugar in general and all products that contain sugar

Acidifying Alcohol
Beer, hard liquor, spirits, and wine

Other Acidifying Food Products
Cocoa, coffee, soft drinks, vinegar, and mustard

Energy Medicine

Energy medicine uses energy fields to treat illness and to improve the human condition. Widely accepted therapies rely on vibration, wavelengths, and frequencies. These include pulsed fields, magnetic fields, alternating current (AC) and direct current (DC) fields, laser, and visible light.

☯ PEMF, PULSED ELECTRO-MAGNETIC FIELD THERAPY

We not only need food, water, sunlight, and air to live but also the natural magnetic signals of the earth. They are very important for the internal regulation of the body.

Not only has the Earth's magnetic field decreased over the last 400 years, but the Earth's signals have also become very distorted by our technological lifestyle. Electrical appliances, mobile phones, satellite signals, power grids, broadcast stations, asphalt, drainage pipes—all of these are responsible.

Unfortunately, our immune system suffers.

Magnetic fields move through the body freely as if it wasn't there—even the bones are essentially transparent. The body uses these fields to generate more cellular energy. This increased energy is needed to help the body heal and regain balance. Healthful magnetic fields are a key in supporting an effective immune response and a healthy overall body.

PEMF therapy has the following positive effects on your body:

- Improved micro-circulation
- Increased supply of oxygen, ions, and nutrients to cells
- Increased partial oxygen pressure
- Increased ATP production by excitation of electrons
- Stimulation of DNA and RNA production

- Accelerated protein bio-synthesis by electron and energy transfer
- Anti-oxidation regulation with increased circulation of available electrons
- Increased calcium transport and absorption for stronger bones, joints, and muscles
- Enhanced cellular tissue elasticity with increased collagen production
- Stimulation of cellular repair mechanism
- Accelerated detoxification of cells and organs
- Decreased swelling, inflammation, and pain
- Boosting of the immune system
- Supporting the body's internal self-regulating mechanisms by activating cellular and molecular processes.
- Stimulates the release of endorphinsThe increased efficiency of toxic removal is only possible by restoring your body's optimal mitochondrial energy so that mercury, lead, dioxin, and PCB can be successfully excreted out of your body.

> *"Disruption of electromagnetic energy in cells causes impaired cell metabolism. This is the final common pathway of disease. If cells are not healthy, the body is not healthy," says Dr. William Pawluk, MD.*

Pulsed Electro-Magnetic Field Therapy has been accepted in many countries.

Dr. Garry Gordon, in Payson, Arizona, incorporated PEMF therapy in his FIGHT program, as did Dr. Anderson in Humlegarden, Denmark, and Dr. Douwes in Bad Aibling, Germany.

To find a PMT-100 practitioner in your local area, please contact NuBioMag at info@pemf.us

☯ SOUND ENERGY THERAPY

Sound energy therapy, also called vibrational energy, uses different modules to create sound frequencies—for example, Tibetan bowls or tuning forks. Certain healing frequencies resonate within the body to promote healing.

Music is another type of sound energy therapy. Listening to music has been proven to lower blood pressure and to reduce pain and anxiety.

☯ LIGHT THERAPY OR COLOR THERAPY

Color is simply light of varying wavelengths. Light and color are also a form of energy that can promote healing.

☯ RIFE THERAPY

Rife therapy is a vibrational energy that uses ultrasound technology (electrical resonance) to kill bacteria, viruses, fungi, parasites, protozoa, and other pathogens.

There are many rife machines on the market which claim to work like the original one built by Dr. Royal Rife. Be advised that not all of them do!http://www.electrodetox.com/royal-rife-video.php

☯ ZAPPER BY DR. HULDA CLARK

The zapper is a device invented by Dr. Clark. It electrically kills parasites, bacteria, viruses, molds, and fungi.

In her book *The Cure and Prevention of all Cancers*, Dr. Clark states that she has seen no side effects on blood pressure, mental alertness, or body temperature. It has never produced pain although it has often stopped pain instantly.

The zapper uses a 30 KHz frequency at a voltage of about 5 volts which can be felt by all parts of the body.

For more information go to: http://www.drclark.net.

There are many machines on the market that use bioresonance as a form of therapy. Many are used by the clinics we visited in conjunction with their cancer protocol.

Acupuncture is also a form of energy medicine. It is a well known and successful therapy for treating chronic diseases.

Joy Of Living

☯ BALANCE

No matter what you do, if it gets out of balance, it becomes a burden to the system. Even riding a bike can be detrimental to your health if it is done excessively.

There should be a healthy balance in everything you do. If you can find this balance, you can relax and live life easier. This does not mean you shouldn't exhaust yourself while participating in sports. On the contrary, sport is a great physical activity. But afterwards, you need to have an adequate time for rest and recovery. Both sides to physical exertion are equally important.

This balance is important for all areas of life. A busy housewife is often tempted to neglect her own needs in favor of others; this is not good. Take some time to enjoy your passion—whatever it is. A warm magnesuim bath is great way to relax and find your inner peace.

☯ SLEEP

In a complete healing program we should also look at our bedroom because a very good night's sleep is what our body needs to replenish itself from the day. It needs to rest in order to function properly and to repair itself. The immune system is the first to suffer from sleep deprivation. Not getting enough sound sleep can take a devastating toll on your physical body and mind. Cancer, heart disease, diabetes, and obesity have all been reported in recent studies concerning the lack of sleep.

So cleaning up our bedroom can have an immense effect on our sleep.

What shall we look for?

First of all, your bedroom should be a room used only for sleeping, meditation, relaxation, yoga, reading, etc.

It should not be used as a workplace or for watching TV, and your computer should not be in your bedroom. These activities are not only stressful at times and loaded with emotions, but they also have EMFs (electromagnetic fields), which should be strictly avoided in a bedroom.

A good mattress is very important to obtaining restful sleep. Try to avoid coiled mattresses as the metal coils interfere with your electromagnetic field. There are great alternatives on the market, but an organic latex mattress or organic wool mattress would be our recommendation.

Opt for cotton linen sheets (preferably organic cotton) as all synthetic fibers such as nylon, polyester, and acrylic are made of thermoplastics and, therefore, off-gas plastic molecules whenever they are heated.

More than likely, all polyester-cotton blends are treated with formaldehyde. Polyester is also manufactured with antimony, a carcinogen that is toxic to the heart, lungs, liver, and skin.

Always wear comfortable cotton nightwear that has not been treated with brominated flame-retardants. Also make sure your pajamas fit properly and are not too small because this restricts the drainage of your lymphatic system.

Get fresh air into your bedroom every day. Air from outdoors is usually better than the air from a closed-up house. Fresh oxygen is very beneficial for a good night's sleep.

❧ LAUGHTER

Laughing is one of the best cures for the heart and soul; unfortunately, this simple remedy has been forgotten. Even a simple smile is difficult for many because of their worries and stress.

You can either watch a funny video (Oliver Hardy and Stan Laurel) or you can go to a laughter yoga group. Learn to laugh again by reading jokes or watching funny cartoons, and train your face to smile again.

Whenever you are trying too hard, it can backfire and have the opposite results. When you try to be extra grumpy, start your day with meanness and growl at everyone you meet. You will soon realize that this feeling has turned around, and you can hardly keep from smiling.

☯ LEISURE TIME

Not everyone is blessed with the opportunity to do what they love and to love what they do. Most of us are required to work in a field or trade that is not our first choice, and it's exhausting. No matter how well you perform your duties, it still makes you tired. That's why it is extremely important to find a balance by doing what you love to do. You must find the time for things you enjoy, like reading a book, listening to music, painting a picture, creating a sculpture, or any other activity that you are passionate about. No matter what your passion is, DO IT. Find the time to engage the mind with something that inspires and uplifts you.

☯ DANCING / MUSIC

You don't need to take lessons to enjoy the healing benefits of dancing. Just swing and sway to your favorite song. Dancing has a very powerful effect on your lymph system, and it helps you detox, gets your heart pumping, activates your adrenal glands, and makes you happy. Start out slowly and gradually increase your rhythm and body movements.

A great way to do this is on a rebounder to some pop music that inspires you to move more. It's a great exercise and helps you on many levels.

Medical Treatments

Laboratory Testing

It is very wise—and highly recommended—to test your blood, saliva, urine, and stool for deficiencies, toxins, and parasites. This helps you establish a list of priorities based on what you need most.

There are many different tests on the market, but we have only listed those that are not always common in orthodox medicine. It is very important to understand that no one should rely on any one test because some test results can have a false positive or false negative result.

☯ TUMOR MARKER TESTS:

A tumor marker is a substance produced by cancer cells; therefore, it is found at higher levels in people with cancer.

Tumor markers can be found even when the tumor is too small to be detected.

Some of the tumor markers are:

- CA-15.3 for breast cancer
- CA- 19.9 for pancreatic, bile duct, colon, and stomach cancers
- CA-125 for cancers of the reproductive system including uterus, fallopian tubes, and ovaries
- S-100 for malignant melanomas
- CEA for colon cancer
- HCQ for testicular cancer
- EVP for nasophyryngeal cancer
- Alpha fetoprotein (AFP) often elevated in liver cancers

- PSA prostate specific antigen for prostate cancer

☯ HCQ URINE TEST

This is a cancer-screening test that detects cancer cells even before signs or symptoms develop. The human chorionic gonadotropin hormone is measured as a detection of cancer or as an indicator of the effectiveness of a specific mode of therapy. The test is very cheap; therefore, it can be repeated very often. http://navarromedicalclinic.com/

☯ CHEMOSENSITIVITY TESTING

This is a test to determine which drugs are the best treatment, the intermittent drugs, and the ineffective drugs for your particular type of cancer. This test is mandatory prior to chemotherapy to determine if this treatment has the potential to work or not.

The cancer cells are harvested out of the blood, genetically broken down, and tested on markers that are compatible with your treatment.

There are only two worldwide laboratories that do the test with blood.

Biofocus Institute for Laboratory Medicine, 45659 Recklinghausen, Germany. Contact: Dr. Lothar Prix +49 2361-3000-130 or e-mail: prix@biofocus.de

Download the brochure here: http://www.biofocus.de/PDF/Onkologie/BF_111_Brochure_M-Oncology.pdf

Research Genetic Cancer Centre, Florina, Greece. Call +30-24630-42264 or e-mail: jpapasot@doctors.org.uk

☯ DARKFIELD MICROSCOPY

This test enables doctors to view living blood cells under a darkfield microscope. Depending on how the cells look, they judge how healthy the cells are. Additional lab tests can then be performed to provide a more comprehensive clinical picture of an individual's condition.

☯ THERMOGRAPHY OR THERMAL IMAGING

This test is mostly used for breast cancer but can also be used with whole body imaging. An infrared camera capable of scanning is used to measure the body surface temperature and detect any signs of inflammation. It is very reliable, non-invasive, non-toxic, and not painful.

☯ LIVER TESTS

These tests include albumin, alkaline phosphatase, alanine transaminase (ALT or SGPT), aspartate transaminase (AST or SGOT), total bilirubin, total protein, LDH, total globulin, albumin/globulin ratio, and GGT.

☯ LIPID TESTS

This is a group of simple blood tests that reveal important information about the types, amount, and distribution of the various types of fats (lipids) in the bloodstream. It includes total cholesterol, HDL (good) cholesterol, LDL (bad) cholesterol, risk ratio (good to total), and triglycerides.

☯ VITAMIN D-25-HYDROXY BLOOD TEST

This test rules out any vitamin D deficiency.

☯ CYTOKINE BLOOD TEST

Cytokines modulate the inflammatory response. The test detects the level of inflammation in your body.

☯ VITAMIN B12, FOLATE BLOOD TEST

As vitamin B12 and folate are derived solely from dietary intake such as eggs, beef, poultry, and fish, many people are deficient in these important vitamins. They play an important role in energy levels, muscle strength, and memory. The blood test will help your doctor diagnose central nervous disorders, anemia, and malabsorption syndromes.

☯ C-REACTIVE PROTEIN TEST

The C-reactive protein blood test measures the level of systemic inflammation. Inflammation is the common denominator of all chronic diseases.

☯ CANDIDA ANTIBODIES BLOOD TEST

This candida test is able to detect systemic candidiasis, which means wherever there is a candida infection (mouth, vagina, or GI tract), this test will find it. Candida, as mentioned in an earlier chapter, will continually weaken and poison our bodies.

☯ COMPREHENSIVE METABOLIC PROFILES

This test provides you a thorough biochemical assessment of your health. Included in it are basic cardiovascular tests, liver and kidney tests, complete blood counts, lipid (fat) tests, diabetes test, mineral tests (total iron, calcium and phosphorus), thyroid test, and fluid and electrolyte tests. The comprehensive metabolic profile test can vary slightly depending on the laboratory.

☯ SALIVA HORMONE TEST

Hormones are key messengers between the brain and the body. When the brain needs something done, it uses hormones to communicate the command to the target organ. Without hormones, the body is unable to effectively repair and regenerate itself, which leads to old, dysfunctional cells.

Saliva is an ideal diagnostic medium to measure the bioavailable levels of steroid hormones active in the tissue. It is this fraction of the total hormones that is free to enter the target tissues in the brain, uterus, skin, and breasts.

Hormones tested in saliva are

estradiol (E2) / estrone (E1) / estriol (E3) / progesterone (pg) / testosterone (T) / DHEA-S (Ds) / cortisol (C).

☯ THYROID BLOOD TEST

The thyroid is the organ that controls your metabolism; therefore, it controls every cell in your body. The thyroid hormones are an important part of the perfect functioning of your body. Testing these hormones is mandatory to eliminate all the causes as to why your body is not functioning properly.

☯ IODINE BLOOD TEST

Iodine plays an important role in hypothyroid conditions and breast cancer. To find out if you have enough iodine, a simple urine iodine test is of high value.

☯ FOOD SENSITIVITY PROFILES AND ALLERGY TESTING

Many health issues are related to food sensitivities. They can cause inflammation, leaky gut, and many undesirable symptoms. Eliminating these foods from your diet is a critical component of any comprehensive approach to health. This test measures your sensitivity to certain foods from an antibody mediated immune response. The antibodies IgG are measured in this test.

☯ HEAVY METAL TESTING

Some laboratories that perform these tests can be found on this website:

http://americanmetaboliclaboratories.net/ They offer a "Cancer Profile Test" and the "Longevity Profile Test ," which is called a biochemical full body scan.

http://lef.org

http://www.zrtlab.com

http://directlabs.com

http://www.metametrix.com/

Metronomic Treatments

Continuous or frequent treatment with low doses of anticancer drugs, often given with other methods of therapy, is called metronomic treatment. This can be done with low-dose chemotherapy but also with natural, anti-cancer drugs.

The most frequently used anti-cancer drugs in metronomic treatments are the following:

☯ LOW DOSE NALTREXONE

Naltrexone is a synthetic drug similar to morphine that blocks opiate receptors in the nervous system and is primarily used in the treatment of heroin addiction.

Low dose naltrexone might exert its effects on tumor growth through a mix of three possible mechanisms:

> By inducing increases of metenkephalin (an endorphin produced in large amounts in the adrenal medulla) and beta endorphin in the blood stream;By inducing an increase in the number and density of opiate receptors on the tumor cell membranes, thereby making them more responsive to the growth-inhibiting effects of the already-present levels of endorphins, which induce apoptosis (cell death) in the cancer cells; andBy increasing the natural killer (NK) cell numbers and NK cell activity and lymphocyte activated CD8 numbers, which are quite responsive to increased levels of endorphins.

PubMed http://www.ncbi.nlm.nih.gov/pubmed/6300232?dopt =Abstract

More information at http://www.lowdosenaltrexone.org/index.htm

☯ DICLOROACETIC ACID

The Michelakis team reports that DCA, dicloroacetic acid, turns on the mitochondria of cancer cells, allowing them to commit cellular suicide, or apoptosis.

Cancer cells shut down the mitochondria, which is the part of the cell that is involved in metabolism and, incidentally, initiates the cell suicide.

A non-cancerous cell will initiate apoptosis when it detects damage within itself that it cannot repair. But a cancer cell resists the suicide process.

Michelakis and his team discovered that they could re-activate the mitochondria of cancer cells. Not only that, but DCA is very effective in doing it. To quote from the Michelakis paper: "The decrease in [Ca2+]i occurs within 5 [minutes] and is sustained after 48 [hours] of DCA exposure." The mitochondria are so sensitive to DCA that just five minutes of exposure reactivates them for 48 hours.

Refer to: http://www.thedcasite.com

☯ BOSWELLIC ACID (PRIOR TO AND DURING LOW-DOSE CHEMOTHERAPY)

Boswellic acid is found in a resinous extract from the Boswellia carteri tree, traditionally used in Ayurvedic medicine as an anti-inflammatory agent. Boswellia acid is an inhibitor of a specific enzyme (5-lipoxygenase) which is often expressed by many types of cancer. This enzyme generates compounds that have potent growth factor activities for cancer. An inhabitation of this enzyme results in tumor shrinkage and increased cell apoptosis.

❂ CURCUMIN

Curcumin, the potent agent of turmeric, is known to slow growth, promote cell death by apoptosis, and increase responsiveness to chemotherapy drugs in a wide range of clinical studies.

❂ POMEGRANATE JUICE

Researchers at the University of California - Riverside have identified components in pomegranate juice that both inhibit the movement of cancer cells and weaken their attraction to a chemical signal that promotes the metastasis of prostate cancer to the bone.

University of California - Riverside (2010, December 12). "Pomegranate juice components could stop cancer from spreading, research suggests." *Science Daily*. Retrieved October 28, 2011 from http://www.sciencedaily.com /releases/2010/12/101212121741.htm

❂ IPT= INSULIN POTENTATION THERAPY

This therapy was discovered in 1926 by Donato Perez Garcia, MD, and is now fostered by his son and grandson.

What is IPT and how does it work?

☯ INSULIN POTENTIATED THERAPY

Insulin receptors are found in every cell of the body, sitting mainly on the membrane of the cell. Insulin interacts with these receptors and is responsible for the regulation of the absorption of glucose, gene regulation, and tissue growth. Insulin is one of the most basic metabolic and control hormones. Cancer cells have far more insulin receptors on their membrane than normal, healthy cells, and some cancer cells even secrete these hormones themselves, resulting in faster growth. More insulin receptors means more insulin effect; the membrane of the cell gets permeable and lets in more of the glucose.

When a patient fasts for one full day, it causes hypoglycemia (not enough glucose in the blood). Then insulin, combined with the cancer drug, is given intravenously. The hungry cancer cells, which were starved of glucose beforehand, and the cells with the most insulin receptors will immediately grab the insulin and the cancer drug. The insulin changes the permeability of the membrane and the cell readily accepts the drug. The cancer cell can be killed.

This enables the drug to be given in a much smaller dose, making it far less toxic to normal cells while building up lethally toxic concentrations in cancer cells. Thus, the growth mechanism of the cancer cell is used against it in IPT. With this method, patients do not suffer the severe side effects that commonly occur with conventional chemotherapy, such as hair loss, vomiting, fatigue, and depression. Therefore, the quality of a patient's life is significantly improved in comparison to what many patients experience when undergoing a conventional treatment.

IPT treatments are successfully used in many clinics in Mexico, Germany, and the United States.

Fever Therapy

☯ · WHOLE BODY HYPERTHERMIA

When we have a fever, the body is creating its own natural immune response. Dr. Gunes says, "Parents should not medicate immediately as fever trains the immune system to fight any illnesses."

Whole body hyperthermia is different from local hyperthermia. Whole body hyperthermia is a holistic cancer treatment that applies heat throughout the whole body with limited side effects. It enhances the immune system, enabling it to find the tumor cells and attack them. A chemical reaction is created on the wall of the cell by the heat, and the immune system can then find the cell more specifically and easily.

New studies show that when the application is extended from two to three hours to six to eight hours, the treatment will also directly kill the tumor. In the case of metastasis, the blood flow is increased throughout the body; therefore, a targeted response is not as effective, and this whole body process is needed. Whole body hypothermia also helps to bring the chemotherapy inside the cell. Because the blood vessels are weakened, the heat helps the process and simultaneously flushes any chemotherapy waste product from the body, which lowers the side effects of the chemotherapy.

Whole body hyperthermia (WBH) is a new treatment using the well known principle of fever in a therapeutic way. There are different methods of action:

- Fever to activate the immune system
- Heat for thermic damage to cancer tissue
- Thermic increase of the efficiency of chemotherapy

Moderate whole body hyperthermia stimulates the immune system.

Moderate whole body hyperthermia mainly activates the immune system. This treatment is given when chemotherapy is not appropriate. The body core temperature is raised to about **39.5 C,** which simulates a natural fever and causes an increase in the number and activity of natural cells, T-helper cells, and cytotoxic T-cells. This treatment is also used in cancer diseases with special association to the immune system like renal cell carcinoma, malignant melanoma, and special lymphomas.

Moderate whole body hyperthermia is also used to prevent recurrences.

Extreme whole body hyperthermia is used particularly in advanced or metastatic disease.

Extreme whole body hyperthermia is used in combination with chemotherapy in advanced or metastatic cancer. The body core temperature is increased up to **42 C.**

Extreme whole body hyperthermia is useful in advanced cancer, especially with metastases in different organs, such as the liver, bones, or lungs.

Used in conjunction with whole body hyperthermia, chemotherapy is more effective. The protocol starts the chemotherapy at a temperature of about 41 C. Very often it is possible to use very low doses of chemotherapy so that side effects of the chemotherapy are kept to a minimum. Tumors or metastases resistant to chemotherapy can be successfully treated with a combination treatment of high doses of vitamin C and whole body hyperthermia.

The body's core temperature is increased carefully using water filtered infrared-A-irradiation. Extreme whole body hyperthermia is a safe treatment.

During whole body hyperthermia, the patient is in a special unit and can be reached from all sides.

☯ LOCAL HYPERTHERMIA

Hyperthermia is an application used to heal cancer by pointedly raising the temperature in the tumor tissue. Thanks to modern technology, this can be done without causing any harm to the patient. With the help of an applicator, short waves are sent into the tumor and damage it.

Unlike classical radiation where X-ray radiation is used, the microwaves are not radioactive. Therefore, this therapy is applicable to most patients for healing cancer, regardless of tumor stage and general condition. Also, the immune system is not destroyed or even disturbed by the use of these waves, which means a much faster recovery.

At a certain temperature range, the destruction of the tumor is initiated without harming healthy tissue. This effect is due to the ability of healthy cells to conduct away the artificial heat faster and more effectively; most tumors lack this ability. As a consequence, very high temperatures are accumulated in the tumor cells, which lead to their destruction by the natural scavenger cells of the body.

The effect of hyperthermia is particularly high for solid tumors, the recurrence of previously treated tumors (relapse), and metastases.

Nowadays, many scientists classify hyperthermia as the fourth column against cancer. Its effect has been well studied in large university centers in Europe and Japan. There are more than 20,000 completed hyperthermia studies related to cancer.

Local hyperthermia is particularly suitable for localized and deep-seated tumors and metastases, such as:

- Thoracic and abdominal cancer
- Lung and liver tumors and/or metastases
- Gastro-intestinal and bladder cancer
- Brain tumors
- ENT tumors
- Lymph node metastases and localized lymphoma

- Sarcomas of all types
- Prostate cancer
- Bone cancer and bone metastases
- Skin cancer

In almost every German cancer clinic, we were introduced to ONCOTHERM Local Hyperthermia as a holistic cancer treatment. We had the pleasure of interviewing the founder-inventor, Prof. Dr. András Szász at the Oncology Congress at Baden, to give you a deeper understanding of just how this treatment works.

http://www.canceriscurablenow.tv/newsletter/german-miracle-cure
http://www.canceriscurablenow.tv/newsletter/hyperthermia-dleted-scene

☯ VIRAL FEVER THERAPY

There are many world-renowned cancer clinics using fever therapy as part of their protocol to heal cancer. A fever is the body's highly evolved attempt to destroy invading organisms and to sweat impurities out through the skin. Fever is an effective, natural process for curing disease and restoring health. Hypocrites, the founder of Western medicine, said more than 2,000 years ago, "Give me the power to create a fever, and I shall cure any disease."

Induced or naturally occurring fever achieves the following:

During a fever, the functionality of the immune system is stimulated, while the growth of bacteria and viruses are forced to slow down. The production of white blood cells, the primary agents of the immune system, is increased as is the rate of their release into the blood stream. The generation of antibodies speeds up as does the production of interferon, an antiviral protein that also has powerful cancer-fighting properties.

A few of the clinics we visited administer active fever therapy generated by a viral infection. The fever activates the immune system dramatically and also creates heat shock proteins on the surface of cancer cells. This effect makes the cancer visible and vulnerable to the increased number of immune cells. The increased blood flow and oxygenation during the process helps to detoxify the body at the same time.

Gene Manipulation

As we have learned from epigenetics, there is a trigger for turning on genes. This means that it's not relevant that you have inherited a cancer gene from your family, but it is important that you do not pull the trigger.

The problem is that we not only inherit the genes but also the lifestyle. We live in the same environment our parents did; we absorb the same toxins; we eat the same food; we share their opinions, likes, and dislikes; and we mimic their physical tendencies.

And that's what triggers those genes. Speaking with Dr. Burzynski, we learned that there are many triggers in epigenetics. Certain foods can trigger certain genes. Even thoughts and emotions can be triggers. Lifestyle is a trigger in a very big way!

So how can you influence that?

Don't follow in the footsteps of your parents and make the same mistakes as they did. It's that simple.

Foods are very active epigenetic triggers, and if you eat natural foods, you activate a lot of tumor suppressor genes. If you think balanced and kind thoughts, you activate them as well.

☯ ANTINEOPLASTONS

Antineoplaston treatment is an experimental therapy offered by the Burzynski Clinic, currently available only within clinical trials.

Antineoplastons (ANP) are peptides and amino acid derivatives. Dr. Burzynski was the first to identify naturally occurring peptides in the human body that control cancer growth. He observed that cancer patients typically had a deficiency of certain peptides in their blood as compared to healthy individuals.

According to Dr. Burzynski, antineoplastons are components of a biochemical defense system that controls cancer without destroying normal cells.

The clinical trials encompass a variety of brain tumors in both children and adults. Over the last ten years, more than 2,000 patients have participated in these trials on antineoplastons. Only patients eligible to enroll in clinical trials may receive antineoplaston treatment under study.

To date, ineligible patients may receive approval to enroll from the FDA on an individual basis. Clinical trials (also clinical research, clinical studies) are research studies conducted to determine whether experimental treatments, or new ways of using known therapies, are safe and effective. Carefully conducted clinical trials are necessary to find treatments that work in people and ways to improve health.

As with any treatment, there is a 30 percent probability that the treatment will work. Results can be tested before you start because of genetic screening. In the Burzynski Clinic, every patient is tested, and if the antineoplastons are effective, a treatment can be booked.

Unfortunately, Dr. Burzynski does not focus much on anything else while a patient is in his clinic. Diet, supplementation, and detox are minimally addressed, and no changes are made to a person's lifestyle. It's a bit like, "buy a miracle drug and come back for more if the cancer comes back." I guess this is the price if a clinic grows big and has a rather scientific focus.

Combination Treatments

None of the clinics we visited rely on one therapy alone but combine many of them to achieve the maximum outcome. In fact, that's where the success comes from.

Cancer grows quickly. Once it reaches a critical level, you need to use every available treatment to get ahead of it. It's not possible to work with pancreatic enzymes alone. It's not possible to rely on chemo alone.

Many of the treatments also support each other and so increase their effectiveness. When a clinic uses high doses of vitamin C for instance, after having oxygenated the tumor with ozone, the vitamin C is going to produce oxidation within the tumor, destroying it very similarly to chemotherapy but without any of the side effects.

Some of the most important combinations are the following:

☯ HYPERTHERMIA

With Low-dose Chemo and IPT

This is a standard treatment in Germany. All holistic clinics use this combination. The only difference we found is in the percentage of the chemo agent used. Depending on the patient and how well the patient reacts to the chemo agent, 20 to 50 percent seems to be the norm.

The IPT by itself is a bit controversial. Some doctors say it works well, and they have good results, while others think the results are not as dramatic. The discussion is very simple. Insulin opens the doors of the cancer cells and makes them hungry for sugar. They starve and want to grab every bit of sugar that floats through the body. This part is agreed upon. Now the sugar is introduced at the same time as the chemotherapy, which could mean the cancer cells absorb the chemo agent at the same time as the sugar, but this is where some doctors disagree. The chemo agent has a different molecular structure and is, therefore, not really the right fit for the sugar receptors on cancer cells.

So, by itself, there is some doubt that IPT really has such a dramatic effect, but in combination with hyperthermia it's not as relevant. The sugar, with or without the chemo agent, is now all gobbled up by the tumor. When heat is applied, the cancer cell swells up and cannot breath any more, which leads to a fermentation process in the tumor that kills it from the inside out.

With High Dose Vitamin C

There are many tests that enable you to check if your tumor is reactive to certain chemotherapy drugs but also to natural remedies. If your cancer, for example, is very reactive and can be killed by high doses of vitamin C, you can combine hyperbaric oxygen with high doses of vitamin C and then use hyperthermia to boost the effects.

Cancer cells love sugar and especially fructose; anything with similar attributes will be consumed by the tumor. Vitamin C is one of the substances that is immediately absorbed by the cancer. This is a vital mistake for the cancer. The combination of oxygen and vitamin C creates hydrogen peroxide, which has an apoptotic effect on the cancer cell.

If this combination is supported by heat, which creates an enormous blood supply, and further supported by intense oxygenation, the cancer cell has very little chance to survive.

If this process is repeated several times, the cancer begins to disintegrate, and the high dose of vitamin C turns from killing agent into a cleansing agent. It's hard to believe that such a cheap substance combined with heat and oxygen can have such a lethal effect on cancer without any negative side effects.

With Homeopathic

Some clinics have achieved super results in combining heat and increased blood supply with homeopathy. This is sometimes used when the patient is not responsive to chemo or when the body is already so poisoned that no further drug can be used.

These combinations, with a moderate form of hyperthermia, activate the immune system and detoxify and boost the self-healing mechanism of the body.

Hyperbaric Oxygen and High Dose Vitamin C

We all know from the movie that hyperbaric oxygen plays a vital part in a well-designed cancer treatment and that it intensifies the effects of vitamin C manifold. Combined with hyperthermia, this combo works even better because the body is already primed.

- Again, the benefits of combining ozone with other treatments are the following:
- Hyper-oxygenation
- Pre-conditioning for oxidative therapies
- Immune stimulation
- Invasive dilation

This way, tumors can be more prone to respond to any anti-tumor therapy that is used.

Surgery

☯ BULK REMOVAL

Most doctors confirm that it is best to surgically remove a large tumor of any kind because it would immediately debunk the tumor load, reduce the burden from the body, and free blocked pathways.

Because of the risk of spreading, the same is not true for small tumors. As soon as a cancer tumor is cut, there are billions of cancer cells set free in the body to float in the blood and to reestablish in many different places.

The same rule applies to biopsies. Once the tumor is injured, which can be done even by a needle, the cancer will spread.

Therefore, if the tumor is small, you should try to change the milieu in the body and help your own self-defense mechanism to reduce the load.

The worst thing you can do, in my opinion, is to have chemo or radiation right after surgery as this will weaken your immune system and the floating cells can re-establish and grow.

Chemo, as well as radiation, is known to knock out your immune system for up to half a year.

CHAPTER 3

Experience

There are many great hints we can learn from those who have walked the path before us, and that's what we do in this chapter.

Another important factor is that many countries have particular limitations and, because of that, have developed strengths in other areas.

The United States, for example, cannot make use of ozone and hyperthermia; therefore, it has focused on supplements and dietary concepts with great success.

Germany, to the contrary, relies strongly on their machinery and therefore ignores dietary concepts greatly.

In this book you will find all those treatments which work with great success in all countries, which means you can build your own treatment plan without limitations.

Caution

☯ FANATICS

Everybody who claims to have found a cure and tries to sell it to you is certainly not your **partner**. There are a lot of remedies that help, but they are not cures. Many of them work for about 10 to 30 percent of the people who try them, but you should never rely on them. It's well worth it to test these remedies and see how they influence the healing process, but without changing the milieu of the body, supplementing the deficiencies, detoxifying the system, and clearing your emotional mess, NO remedy will ever help.

Many of the people who find these remedies very successful also report that it is a never-ending battle because the cancer keeps coming back in other places.

Black salve, for instance, is a good example of that. We interviewed a patient who has used and advertised this product very convincingly. She has cured many of her own melanomas only to find others emerging in new places. Today, four years later, she is no closer to being cancer-free and is quite possibly in worse condition than when she started using the salve.

IF YOU DO NOT REMOVE THE CAUSE, YOU CANNOT CURE CANCER!

☯ CHARLATANS

Big promises are very attractive but seldom true. In the past four years we have followed many of these promises and have not found an ounce of evidence that they hold true. The problem is that cancer has become a big business.

The main reason for such a cancer business boom is that cancer patients all search for a simple and convenient solution. They will buy pretty much anything and everything that promises an easy solution. Just give me a pill so that I can go on with my life.

That's why you will find displays with so-called miracle cures at all health shows and trade fairs. Just drink this juice or this water, or use this ointment, and your cancer will disappear. Or, you read headlines like THIS TREATMENT MELTS TUMORS LIKE ICE IN THE SUN. They are all false claims to extract money from you.

We would let you know if we had found such a miracle treatment, but we have not.

☯ NARROW MINDED

It does not matter if you speak to a homoeopathist who tells you to ONLY use his medicine or an oncologist who tells you to stay away from IV treatments and supplements. Anybody who excludes other treatments is a fanatic.

These people are not your partner. Cancer is a multi-faceted disease and can be approached from many angles. You never know what works best in individual situations or which combination does the trick. You need to include all elements of the body, mind, and spirit. In many cases, one treatment supports the next.

Many of the clinics we visited have a treatment protocol that offers a variation of three to ten treatments, all complementing each other.

The easiest way to evaluate your doctor's advice is whether or not he supports all of the mandatory treatments we listed in Chapter 2. If he tells you to stay away from these treatments . . . RUN!

And, as Charlotte Gerson said, "Don't argue. Just walk out and never come back. Arguing will only cost you energy, which you can use in other places more effectively."

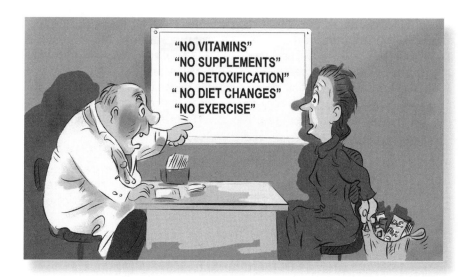

☯ SHARKS

Cancer can be directly translated into $$$$$$$. You are like a wounded animal and many sharks will circle around you. They smell money like a shark smells blood.

On our journey we met a lot of practitioners who are in it for the money. They prescribe for you what makes them the most $$$, not what you need most. They rush you into treatments that might never have been your first choice if you had known what your options were and what you really needed.

In the alternative health market you will find hundreds of claims for successful cancer treatments and diagnostic tools—from energy healing to crystals to magnets—all working wonders. I especially love the high tech, computer-generated quantum and love waves. They sell like hotcakes and have absolutely no effect whatsoever, besides the placebo effect. They are money-making machines to sell you nothing but hot air.

Here is a hint that is absolutely accurate—if they offer you these high tech diagnostic tools, those quantum readers and laser DNA testers to lay your hand on for a health diagnosis, they are trying to sell you science fiction. These machines can NOT reproduce the same results when you use them five minutes later. Ask your doctor to do the test again under a different name. If they say it's not possible . . . WALK AWAY. They are all a hoax and, believe me, it's not only you who falls prey to their big sales pitch. Clinics and doctors also buy this rubbish and offer it to their patients because it sells. And it costs YOU money! Health diagnostic tools have to be accurate and results have to be reproducible, otherwise they don't count. Random results are not what you want.

According to Voll, Electro-Acupuncture is a very accurate tool to diagnose allergies, deficiencies, and all other energy-related tests. The results are always accurate and may vary from practitioner to practitioner slightly, but they are never random.

In our documentary, "CANCER is curable NOW," we have investigated and filtered through all of the different treatment options and only focus on the ones that really work. However, it's very important for you to check it yourself.

Are the diagnostic tools or treatments successful against cancer and where is the evidence?

We have seen chiropractors offer anti-cancer treatment even though there is no evidence, whatsoever, that the alignment of a spine has anything to do with healing cancer. We have seen reiki masters treat cancer patients without advising the patient to do all the other things that would be necessary, and probably much more effective, and so the patients die. In fact, this is the reason the alternative branch of healers has such a bad name.

There is so much ignorance, narrow-mindedness, and greed in the healing business that it's really hard for an uneducated patient to survive.

I do believe that these practitioners can play an important role in your healing and that they are helpful in the process, but in the right hierarchy. Some things are more important than others. It would be a pity if you spent your money and had nothing left for where it's needed most.

☯ HIDDEN COSTS

Many patients are often very intimidated by a doctor and are not brave enough to ask in detail about the costs involved to get them well. Others are so impressed by the certainty of a doctor and believe that he is only concerned about their health that they trust blindly without asking for a quote. Both types of patients are usually in for a very tough wake up call.

Doctors are no saints. They charge money, and if you don't have any, they won't treat you. If you run out of money before the treatment is finished, they send you home.

We have spoken to many patients, and most of them pay a small fortune on top of their quoted fees due to the small print or extra treatments that had not been quoted. This adds tension, which you do not need. In fact, stress is unhealthy.

So check into all the details before you start. Don't let them deceive you with a quote which is covering only the basics and then they add many more procedures, treatments, tests, and other expenses along the way.

Ask for a detailed quote for the proposed treatment, and talk to the doctor about your financial status. Tell them honestly how much you have to spend so that they don't plan way beyond your budget. Make sure you are spending your money on necessities and with your priorities in mind.

Also, discuss the value of the different treatments with one or more doctors before you start. Some treatments have a minimal effect, and others are absolutely mandatory. Do what's necessary in the clinic and then follow up as an outpatient. You don't need an expensive room when you can do most things in the comfort of your own home.

Money is a great asset to have when you get sick. Don't waste it. Keep it tight and invest it wisely.

☯ BARGAIN FOR YOUR LIFE

We have met patients who have actually bargained before they started treatment and guess what? Some have received treatment with a 30 percent discount over others.

In a Mexican clinic, we spoke to a group of patients while they sat in the IV room and found out that some of them had shopped around at all the different clinics prior to starting treatment. They found prices ranging between $100 and $300 per one ozone therapy; so don't be afraid to ask. Do some research and find a way to fit what you need into your budget. Call different clinics and bargain for your life.

Check Your Doctor

☯ RECORDING

Not all doctors will like it, but you should request a recording of what he or she said to you. Or take your phone and record the conversation yourself.

There are three main reasons why you need to make this mandatory. The first one is that you are not able to absorb everything they say in a short consultation. You just won't.

Our minds are trained to recognize things we know and have been familiarized with. It's like walking through a shopping mall; you will only see what is in your field of awareness, and everything else will pass by unnoticed. My wife, for example, would never see a new Mac on display while I would never see a sale on schoolbooks for our kids. We hear and see what we are familiar with.

The second reason to record every conversation with your doctor is to be able to listen again and again until you understand what he or she said. When I listened to the recordings of the interviews, I heard so much more than I did during the actual interview. It's because your mind gets used to the music, as Dr. Gordon mentioned in our interview. There is a lot of new vocabulary and jargon that needs to be learned in order to understand it.

And the third reason is to hold your doctor accountable. He is less likely to say something careless if he knows he is being recorded. This will cause them to be careful about the words they choose and the manner in which they express themselves.

We have learned that when a patient requests to record the consultation for future reference, they receive more respect and are treated more carefully. The doctor does not attempt to rush them into unnecessary treatments in a "hush-hush" manner. The doctors feel more accountable for the advice they give.

Now, let's just say your doctor will not allow you to record the conversations. There is a very simple and mandatory solution.

Go somewhere else.

Don't try to record secretly; that would only defeat the purpose. Don't argue either. You will not win the battle. Just pack your suitcase and leave. There are a million doctors out there, and you only need one who is willing to be accountable for what he says and does!

Be firm—it's your life they are talking about!

☯ SECOND AND THIRD OPINIONS

Just like Dr. Gordon said in the movie, "You need to get used to the music before you understand what you hear." Having a second and even a third opinion from different doctors and faculties will provide you with several different options and viewpoints.

The same issue can be approached from many different sides.

A homeopathic doctor, for example, will always use homeopathic remedies and energy to cure you. A surgeon will always think you have disposable body parts. A medical doctor will prescribe medicine. The herbalist will use herbs and mushrooms and diet to strengthen and detoxify. Every trade offers to solve your problem with their particular expertise.

The danger in that is that they will try to hold you to their truth even though their solution might only be part of the puzzle.

Cancer is one of the most dangerous end stages of a physical break down. Many things must have gone wrong in order to get to this place.

That's why good holistic oncologists do not exclude one treatment over another. They don't try to sell you surgery alone, or chemotherapy and nothing else. Nor do they promise to heal you with homeopathic remedies.

They incorporate everything possible. In many clinics they use homeopathic remedies to stimulate the detox and boost the immune system. They use herbs, juices, diet, and immune boosters. They support you with high dose IV treatments together with sodium bicarbonate, hyperthermia, oxygenation, and surgery (when necessary). They help you find peace and teach you to meditate. They reintroduce you to a loving, caring lifestyle. They teach you how to prepare healthy meals. They give you the knowledge and the tools to handle life.

Holistic means to approach a problem from every angle by treating a patient physically, mentally, and spiritually.

I am not asking you to only trust doctors who provide you with all the different treatments and options. But you need to find one who is open to all of them and incorporates them into the plan. If a doctor has no clue about diet, that's okay as long as he does not negate the issue by telling you it doesn't matter, attempting to deter you from incorporating a healthy and supportive diet into your treatment plan.

☯   ALLOPATHIC / HOLISTIC

There is a need for both, the conventional and the holistic doctor.

Many times your insurance will pay for conventional treatments and tests, but they do not always pay for your alternative holistic doctor. That's why it's wise to have both.

Make use of both systems and get what you need from your conventional doctor paid by your insurance and invest wisely into holistic treatments yourself. If you manage to get your doctor and naturopath and dietitian all working together, it's certainly best, but it's not mandatory.

The key here is to know what you want and then ask for it. Many times you will be able to receive the treatment you need if you inquire at different clinics or treatment centers. We found several clinics in the United States offering the moderate form of hyperthermia. There is no need to fly to Germany if you can have it at your doorstep, but you need to ask for it. You need to become proactive in your healing process. You can also get ozone treatment almost everywhere. We even saw communities that purchased an ozone generator and hired a nurse to do the treatment.

The key here is that you need to research and find what you need.

☯ COMPARE ALL OFFERS

Healing can be dangerous if you have all your eggs in one basket.

You often hear that a patient dies from the treatment and not from the cancer. In 80 percent of all cases, this is a fact. That's why it's so important to have a knowledge-based overview of what you need to do.

For instance, if you use chemo, you not only kill the cancer but you also destroy your immune system. This means that while you are recovering from the so-called cure, you have no defense, and the few remaining cancer cells can literally explode in your body without anything holding them back.

Exactly the same thing happens when you use radiation. You not only destroy the tumor but also all of the surrounding tissue. In doing so, you hinder the healing process and prevent the natural healing reactions of the body. Plus, your immune system is down for a minimum of six months. So where is the benefit in that?

If you go to a clinic where they do everything possible to reduce the tumor size but at the same time they feed you cheese, macaroni, and pudding, you will not benefit from the treatment either. Food that is converted into sugar feeds your cancer, and you negate every treatment, no matter how effective it appears.

Unfortunately, there are NOT a lot of clinics that provide everything as it should be. Some lack the knowledge necessary to educate their patients in the new lifestyle, others lack the dietary programs to support healing, and others lack mental and spiritual components of the healing process.

Unfortunately, 90 percent of all clinics lack the knowledge and integrity towards their patients to incorporate everything possible into their programs. They offer a small portion and don't inform their patients of all other treatments that they have to get somewhere else.

It's actually very rare that you will find everything under one roof. But sometimes you do, and these clinics offer a huge benefit over all others. They remain in charge of your healing process and guarantee a positive outcome.

But let's just say you cannot afford to go to such a clinic. There are ways to create the same environment on your own. You just need to assemble all the pieces to the healing puzzle, determine what needs to be done, and then create a plan of action.

The whole purpose of our education program is to provide you with the knowledge to build a supportive team of practitioners and create a healing environment for yourself.

☯ YOU ARE THE CONTRACTOR

The very first thing you need to understand is that you will always be a victim of ignorance if you can't check if your doctor's advice is actually good or not.

Hiring a doctor who has never actually healed a cancer patient is like hiring a contractor who has never built a house or—even worse—you hire a builder whose houses all break down after a couple of years.

So it's only logical to look at several HOUSES, not builders, to decide whom to hire to build your house. When you find a house you like and you can confirm that it is well built, you can now be confident in the contractor you choose to build your house.

It's no different with doctors. You need to check the patients they have treated and find out if they have had a positive result with their treatment plan. This is what we did when we asked hundreds of patients how they were treated, what worked for them, and which doctor actually helped them to get well. That's what enabled us to find the best of the best. Believe me—we could have interviewed another

1,000 doctors who are successfully assisting their patients in their pursuit of a healthy body. They are everywhere; but to find them you need to know what to look for.

If you are educated and know how to determine if a doctor knows what he is talking about, you will have no problem finding them. But if you don't, the only grounds you can base your healthcare on are faith and trust, which is a huge risk. Believe me, it's a risk you don't want to take. It's worse than Russian roulette with five bullets in a six-chamber gun.

There are a few points to remember:

Don't let them sell you something that does not have a proven success rate in other patients. Ask to speak to the patients. Find out if the patients participated in other treatments at the same time. Often doctors try to sell you a single remedy while they did five at the same time.

Don't let them convince you that you have no other choice. You literally have thousands of options. AND . . .

Don't let them tell you that, based on their statistics, you will die. The only thing their statistics prove is that they have no solution for your problem. Run if that's what they tell you.

☯   WHO FITS YOU BEST!

There are people who have total trust in **modern medicine**. They are probably better off with an oncologist who is open to all other components but still relies on modern scientific research. It's just a better match.

Both the doctor and the patient feel safe.

If you would ask such a doctor to go completely natural, he would feel insecure. In the same way, asking a patient who puts all her trust in modern medicine would feel completely out of place with an all-natural approach. The patient and doctor should be a match in order to feel comfortable and safe.

When we traveled and met different doctors, I could immediately say whom I would trust and whom I would never trust. It was clear because I had learned what I needed to know to judge the doctor according to my values.

You will find the perfect match for yourself in the same manner once you are armed with the knowledge and know the options available to you.

Many times one doctor is the stepping-stone to the next. You learn during the process and evolve. And as you do, you will see that different doctors, different treatments, and different needs will lead you farther down the road to recovery.

NEVER get discouraged and stop learning.

☯ FIND LOCAL SUPPORT

Cancer is not a disease which is healed once and for all and you are over and done with it. Going into a clinic for three weeks is a great start to get you back on track, but it's only the beginning. This healing process requires a lifetime commitment to healthy living and permanent change. That's why you need local support.

Find a team that inspires you, keeps you on track, and holds you to your path when you feel desperate to cheat. We are all habitual beings, and it's very easy for us to slip back to our old life, even if that's what made us sick in the first place.

A good team for a cancer patient would include:

- A diet group for healthy cooking, juicing, and possibly gardeningAn organic market where you buy your locally grown, fresh, organic produce and where, hopefully, you will strike a bargain as a regular customerA fitness group to encourage regular exercise. The little rebounders (mini trampolines) are worth their weight in gold and should be in every group you attend.A local doctor or naturopath for regular IV treatments, checkups, and blood tests. You need to monitor your progress, and you need professional support.

- A learning group for mental input and constant reminders of what's good for you and what's not. You need continuous education. This is where forums, membership groups, and workshops come in. You need them to be reminded over and over again of what you can do to support your healing.

Another key to a bountiful level of life energy is joy and passion. That's why patients need to pursue things they are passionate about in their lives and allow themselves to be magnificent in what they love to do.

Whatever you love doing, whatever you are passionate about, find a local group and join them. Surround yourself with people who share your passion or interests. People do not become friends by accident, but by choice. Surround yourself with passion and share your passion with others.

☯ OVERSEAS SPECIALTY TREATMENTS

There are some worthwhile treatment options that require a journey to a specialist.

In my mind, there would be no question regarding whether to have hyperthermia as part of my healing program. I truly believe in local, as well as whole body, hyperthermia. I would also choose to have ozone therapy but would probably organize that locally. If you go to a foreign clinic anyway, it's usually part of the program, but after you come home, you could continue the ozone treatment locally.

Unfortunately, everybody does not have the money to fly to a clinic overseas and stay there for three to four weeks. That's why we have outlined options in our treatment plan that are mandatory and that come close to the actual treatments. They might not be as effective, but there are options for every budget.

Instead of hyperthermia, for example, you may opt to use an infrared dome or sauna, which also enables you to heat up the body to a fever-like condition. You can take high-dose vitamin C orally before you use the sauna or before you go into a clinic to have hyperbaric oxygen.

Instead of having pharmaceutical angiogenesis inhibitors like Avastin, which has deadly side effects, you can do it naturally together with your diet. You can achieve the same if not better effect with green tea, curcumin, aloe, and over 100 other angiogenesis inhibitors.

There are many ways to simulate those treatments—certainly not to the same extent or the same degree—but you can get close.

IPT, local hyperthermia, and the intense form of hyperthermia always need to be done by experienced doctors and only under professional supervision.

☯ HOW TO FIND THE BEST DOCTOR

This is probably the most frequent question we receive every day. How do I find the best doctor for my needs? How do I know that he or she is the best?

The only way to find out is to know what you are looking for.

In a seminar a little while ago, I learned that the key to hiring a good staff member is a proper job description. The more detailed you describe the job, the more refined your selection will be. You will also be more specific in what you need to know about the person you are looking to hire.

That's why you can't just go to a doctor and ask him to fix you. You need to know what you want from them and then find out if they can provide it.

Our mission is to prepare you for this healing journey. We want you to be in charge of your health. We want you to take responsibility for your life. By taking charge of your health and being responsible for your life, you can only get better.

If you want ozone, you will find a doctor close to you who can treat you. If you look for IV treatments, you will find them.

You are in charge, and if you know the content of this book, you will know what you need.

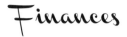
Finances

☯ DESIGN YOUR TREATMENT

A good doctor will design your treatment protocol very carefully so that you have maximum benefit. They plan each treatment in sequence so that they support each other and intensify the healing reaction.

This process is based on experience. If you have the money to purchase all of these treatments in one clinic under the supervision of the same doctor, that's great! But if you don't, book what I call a "designer consultation" and have them prepare a treatment program designed especially for you. This is probably the best investment you can make as it takes the guesswork out of each decision.

A good friend of mine did exactly that and consulted three good oncologists at an early stage of his cancer. Two of the protocols matched almost identically, and the third varied only slightly. Then he searched for all the pieces to the puzzle and tried to gain access at minimal cost. In addition to the medical aspect of his treatment, he complemented the process by following strict dietary guidelines, supplemented well, and exercised a lot.

Only four months after the diagnosis, he was well and his tumor had subsided.

☯ TREATMENT VALUE LIST

The most important step in planning your protocol before you start with any treatment program is a clear evaluation of your assets. If you have plenty of money, you do not need to worry. Just fly to one of the world-renowned clinics and take advantage of everything they have to offer.

If you don't, plan your treatment list carefully.

In the first part of Chapter 2, we thoroughly worked through all of the mandatory treatment options, and you may have already decided which ones feel right for you.

Then, in the first part of Chapter 3, we learned how to work with a doctor to determine the best protocol for you and what you need. You learned to get a second or third opinion and to record everything carefully.

In the second part of Chapter 3, we will help you develop a protocol plan and match it with your budget.

Treatment	Weekly	Location	Cost / Week
Hyperbaric oxygen			$
Supplements			$
IV Zink/ Selenium			$
IV Ozone			$
IV C			$
Organic Veggies			$

Call around and find out what the cost is for everything you will need. Don't forget to write it down for future reference. Get quotes on hyperbaric oxygen. There are many places that offer a 10-pack deal. Find out who offers IV treatments and what it costs. Check into the cost of ozone therapy. It may be a lot cheaper in the long run to buy an ozone generator yourself (under $1,000) and learn how to use it. There are plenty of great books and even workshops to teach you what to do.

If you look carefully, you may even find a doctor near you who offers ozone under the radar. You just need to ask. There are doctors everywhere who actually help their patients, but they like to keep quiet and don't advertise what they do so that they can work in peace. Find them.

Most importantly, plan the treatment according to your needs. If you are full of toxins from your workplace, dental treatments, or vaccinations, then you might want to focus the majority of your efforts and funds on detoxification. You might need several sessions of IV chelation or clay baths or an infrared sauna at your home if that's your main problem.

If you have a lot of emotional stress and can't seem to resolve these issues, you might want to seek help and get your life in order before doing anything else.

If you are deficient and poisoned from dead and toxic food, you might want to supplement via IV treatments and fill up your empty tanks with an all-fresh, organic diet or by following the Gerson protocol.

The priority for your treatment really depends on what your most pressing issues are.

☯ HOLD YOUR MONEY TIGHT

Cancer is not a short-term disease and demands a permanent lifestyle change that requires you to eat the best food and to keep your body well. You will need mountains of supplements for many years—actually right until the end.

There are many patients who get annual healing boosts in Germany or Mexico through a session of hyperthermia or a series of hyperbaric oxygen with IVs. You might need dental treatments from a holistic dentist or a new water filter.

There is so much you will need over time, and it's really important that you plan ahead.

Everything you buy should be long-lasting, good quality, have a purpose, and fit into the healing plan. And if you find a new treatment, research it first, read everything you can find about it, and discuss it in our forums. If you are still convinced that it might help, consult your design doctor to work it into your plan.

No hasty decisions. No need to hurry. You will always have another day when you do things carefully.

☯ DO IT YOURSELF?

Treating yourself and taking charge of the healing process is a bit like flying a plane. Even though you have been a passenger for many years, you have never actually held the steering wheel yourself. To do that NOW in mid-air or shortly before a crash landing is very dangerous.

Rather seek a DOCTOR with experience and have him guide you.

I truly do NOT recommend you to treat yourself as this can backfire.

As you can see from everything we have discussed so far, there are many components to this disease, and it's often very hard to be aware of all of them. If you overlook one important detail, you can spoil everything else you do.

For example, if you are low and deficient in magnesium, all other treatments won't really work. Or if your liver is not working properly, you have now enzymes to help you break down your food. There are a lot of key factors to check, and you can't do that on your own.

As Dr. Anderson said in his interview, "Healing cancer is not a science you learn at school. It is years of experience and dedication. Weeks, months, and years of learning and experimenting will teach you what you need to know in order to help patients."

Please try to find someone with experience and with a passion to help you. They will make your journey more efficient and greatly increase your chances of success.

But there are many things you can do for yourself. In fact, no one else can do them for you.

Clean out the rubbish from your pantry, your bathroom, your fridge, and your living environment. Clean out all the friends who do not inspire you. Stop wasting time on useless things and focus on the essence of life.

Focus on a daily detox program; exercise; drink juices; eat healthy foods; take supplements; practice breathing exercises, yoga, prayer, or meditation; get sound sleep; engage yourself in anything that makes your heart sing.

Dance, sing, play, and enjoy this wonderful world. It's what you are here for.

Learn From Different Sources

☯ CANCER COACHING

If you do not really feel confident to approach this journey towards health all on your own and you do not want to lay all your trust into one single doctor, it's very helpful to look for a cancer coach.

In our movie, we interviewed Bill Henderson and Burton Goldberg, who have both done immense research in the field of holistic cancer treatments.

Burton Goldberg has written several books about alternative cancer treatments and even made a movie called *Cancer Conquest*. He has studied this subject for many years and is now dedicating his life to helping others find their way around. He offers coaching services and knows pretty much every clinic and doctor and their services. His insights are invaluable. ***www.burtongoldberg.com***

Bill Henderson lost his wife to cancer, which was his trigger to study and research alternative treatments. He certainly found the best solutions out there. His best-selling book, *Cancer Free: Your Guide to Gentle, Non-toxic Healing*, which is already in its fourth edition, is a must-read. Bill has created a masterpiece and has helped thousands of patients with his book. Bill also teaches on the radio and with his newsletters. Do sign up. Bill's coaching service can be found on his website. http://www.beating-cancer-gently.com/

There are certainly many more cancer coaches out there who have learned over a long period of time what you have to learn in a rather short time. Make use of their years of experience and have a consultation with them. It will probably save you hundreds of $$$ plus weeks of searching for the right doctor.

☯ WATCH A MOVIE

Reading books is essential, but it's not everybody's favorite thing to do. Plus, when it comes to medical terms, it can be very tiring. That's why there are movies, talk shows, interviews, and radio shows. Learn the way you learn easiest.

In many cases, a video is virtually an effortless way to obtain knowledge and information about any subject. You can learn so much while entertaining yourself. "CANCER is curable NOW" is not the only movie having huge effects on mankind. Watch the "Burzynski Movie," "Knives over Forks," "Foodmatters," "Foodinc," "The Gerson Miracle," "Healing the Gerson Way," "A Beautiful Journey," and so on. There are hundreds of videos that are worth watching. For instance, "Crazy Sexy Cancer" and all the movies from David Getoff are a must-see for everyone.

☯ EVERYTHING ALWAYS HAS TWO SIDES

I know. When you start your research, you will always find something positive and something negative about the same treatment, doctor, or clinic. It's a pain in the butt that these publishers and writers can never be either unanimously for or against a treatment. There is always someone who takes up the opposition.

Everything has two sides.

This is often hard to see, but if you take the time and dig a bit, you will find that everything under the sun has two sides to it—a good one and a bad one. And what you might think is bad for you is good for someone else. For instance, it's good for the cancer industry that there are so many cancer patients, but it's very bad for the individual who gets sick.

Even when you look at cancer from the perspective of a cancer patient, there are good and bad components in the disease. The good aspect of it is that, in order to get well, you have to (finally) resolve all the things that made you sick. You have to change your life for the better in order to get well. This is actually a good thing, which has been confirmed from all of those patients who managed to do it. On the other side, it is hard to accept that this change comes as forcefully as it does. The pain of change is certainly a big issue to overcome.

Good and bad are to be found in everything. Look at people. Take Michael Jackson, for example. Millions hated him for being a pervert and millions loved him for his music. The Dalai Lama has received the Nobel Peace Prize, as a leader involved in war, destruction, and death. He is loved by many and hated by many as well—especially the population in China, which he blamed for this disaster.

George W. Bush is one of my favorite examples. He made a lot of people very rich, and they love him for that. On the other hand, he has millions at his back calling him the devil.

A sports car can be wonderful and great! But if you want to take your six kids to school, it's not a practical choice of transportation. At the same time, a big car will cost more in fuel, and it's hard to find good parking. And we won't even mention the preference in brands!

If I say to my kids, "Broccoli tastes great!" some may agree but certainly not all of them will support my opinion. Even if my children happen to agree, there are many people who hate it. Also, if you eat your favorite food every day and you eat lots of it, you will soon grow to hate it.

It does not matter what you are researching, you will always find opinions that contradict each other—political parties, religions, people, and even computers, like Apple vs. Mac. The pros and cons are represented with equal enthusiasm.

Even within the same community of like-minded people, you will find the same problem. When we spoke to all the doctors and asked about IPT treatments, diet, hyperthermia, or any other treatments, we found some who said that a particular treatment doesn't work and others who praised it as the ultimate treatment, even among the holistic doctors.

The reason for this is that you see everything through the filter of your past experiences. Whatever you have stored in your subconscious mind will determine if an object, person, or situation is good or bad.

For this reason, you need to find your own truth. The more you learn and the more you strive to understand this whole concept of health, the more you will find what works for you.

No one else knows your body like you do. And that's because you live there. And when you learn to listen to that inner voice, you will be well on your way to a speedy recovery.

☯ LEARN FROM THE WEB

There is a lot of information on cancer out there. Unfortunately, most of it is designed to suck you into the system like a vortex. Print media, TV advertising, radio shows, and all the other marketing materials are an attempt to manipulate you and sell you a concept.

Large corporations that make their money by selling their souls to the corporate world own most of the newspapers, magazines, radio channels, and TV stations. They do everything for the $$ and will not stop selling until you refuse to buy. To hope that one day they will give up their monopoly and support you is delusional. They limit all of the information to what they WANT you to know.

A great way to bypass this INFO WAR is the INTERNET. There are so many possibilities for little people like myself, or Mike Adams, Dr. Mercola, Dr. Mark Hyman, Sherrill Sellman, and Dr. Garry Gordon to stir the pot and share what we believe to be the truth.

You can find hundreds of sources that are well presented and well spoken who will share with you how others have overcome this disease.

The great thing is that if you have come this far in reading this book, you are already so well educated that you will not be a victim of any marketing stunt anymore. You are an educated patient who just needs to translate mental knowledge into practical wisdom.

☯ ATTEND WORKSHOPS

There is a great power in community. If you attend workshops and seminars, you actually join a group of like-minded people and the energy propels you forward like nothing else. You get to know new people who all have the same or similar problems as you do.

Groups are formed, and you have a network of people with whom to share your concerns. Many times you will see that people in these groups complement each other. Maybe you meet someone who is good at performing research, while you are better at presenting the findings. Perhaps you will meet someone who has a passion for cooking healthy meals and you enjoy doing the shopping.

Those who conduct workshops usually have a great passion for the subject they speak about. Otherwise they would never go through all of the hard work it takes to plan, schedule, and organize these things. This passion is contagious. It affects you like a virus and starts to bring you into a new field of awareness.

That's why it's great to make it a habit to attend as many seminars and workshops as you can.

CHAPTER 4

Mental Emotional Healing

Methods

There are many methods and techniques available to help a person overcome emotional stress and trauma.

There is:

- Psych K
- EFT (Tapping)
- NLP
- Meditiation
- Pranayama (breathing exercises)
- Mindfulness
- Non-judgment workshops
- The Journey Work
- Beat the Blues
- and many more

Each one of these methods is important to free yourself from feelings that cause you to be sick, and all of them will lead to a calming and understanding of the mind.

Each technique can be a stepping stone to the next, but they will only reveal their true power if you try them. (We will cover all of them in great detail in our COMMON SENSE COMMUNITY FORUM.)

Many of these methods can generate an immediate change in energy, causing you to feel powerful and strong, just like a homeopathic remedy would make you feel by changing your energy vibration. But very often, after a little while, people slip back into their old habits of thought.

The reason for "back-sliding" is that, over the course of your life, most of your emotional patterns are imprinted in your mind with countless layers and repetitions in many situations. When you dissolve one layer, there are still hundreds more to work on. Many of these methods change the symptom but do not actually dissolve the seed/cause of the problem.

Every emotion you feel is driven by a belief. If you do not change the belief, you cannot change the emotion. That's why I personally prefer those methods that work to change your beliefs and imprints.

Any method you choose should become a constant companion. Over time you will become a master at dissolving stress, resentment, jealousy, and any other chronic emotion with a snap of your fingers, but only if you practice.

A good friend of mine uses a simple, yet very powerful technique. When something unfortunate or disturbing happens, he stops and thinks of how he can learn a lesson from this event. He then just says out loud, "NEXT." In his mind, he converts every painful emotion into a lesson on his journey to success and then moves on. He has no time to delve into all the drama because he is too busy moving forward.

We are all on a journey to become a master in all areas of life. There is no reason to be frustrated if we see the challenges, big and small, as lessons along the way. Instead, we see them as opportunities to learn something.

In this chapter, I do not intend to introduce the previously mentioned methods like EFT or meditation and so on, as there are hundreds of teachers close to where you live. I rather encourage you to find a practitioner or group to join so that you can practice these methods and techniques regularly. You can also enjoy a daily session in the convenience of your own home through online courses with stunning communities and exchange possibilities, which will save you a lot of money.

Use common sense in choosing whom to work with.

If you do not feel comfortable in a group and you feel out of place with their ways, move on to the next. This can easily happen. Not every group is in tune with you, nor is every method. Meditation, for example, can be the most wonderful experience in an open-minded community, but it can be a bit weird in a dogmatic, spiritual community which is all about rituals and dress codes.

In the same way, a teacher can be very awkward. I have met some who are stuck in personal issues, fighting with ex-partners, bitter and frustrated, but they are teaching others how to resolve emotional stress. If that's the case, leave silently and search for someone else. There are actually plenty of teachers who have mastered what they teach—find one.

If you feel comfortable in a group and the energy resonates with you, stick to it. You will only get better over time. If at first you don't succeed—try, try again. Imagine that controlling your mind is like ice skating; it takes time to be able to elegantly move over the ice. It requires practice to master any new skill.

Emotional Intelligence

☯   **EVERYTHING IS ENERGY**

> *"What lies behind us and what
> lies before us are small matters
> compared to what lies within us."*
>
> *- Ralph Waldo Emerson*

This first chapter is part of the introduction and a bit technical, but bear with me; it's required to give you a foundation. All else will be easy in comparison.

When we break the universe down into the smallest material particles of existence, we experience a micro cosmos that is as vast as the macro cosmos. The atom, once thought the smallest particle of actual MATTER, contains electrons, neutrons and protons. The distance between the nucleus and the electrons is proportionately as vast as the distance between the earth and the moon. And the electrons are now found to be equally insignificant parts of matter, as they consist of even smaller parts, which hold together by means of magnetism and energy. Only the high speed of movement, which is contained in these tiny forms of energy, forms an apparent material existence.

The amount of energy, which is contained in these atoms, is well known from a nuclear explosion where tiny amounts of matter are set free in a devastating blast.

By mathematical calculation, the amount of energy held in a human body is equivalent to the electricity you need to power all of Las Vegas for a whole month.

At first glance, it can be intellectually challenging to realize that everything in existence is just highly compressed and condensed energy, because we experience matter as a solid, liquid or gas. But this does not change the fact that it's energy vibrating in different frequencies and wavelengths.

This brings us to the concept of Quantum physics.

Though it may seem impossible, energy can be quantified; that is, it can be measured. The unit of measurement is the quantum, which is, by definition, the smallest measurable size of energy. German Scientist Max Planck has defined the dimension of one quantum as 10-35m. He believes this to be the minimum characteristic length that space can have. The total size of our universe from one end to the other (if there are ends to it :-) is roughly 10-26m, depending on how they measure it.

Within these two extremes is our perceived reality with all the things we know.

From these observations, we can conclude that one quantum is the building block from which all things are made.

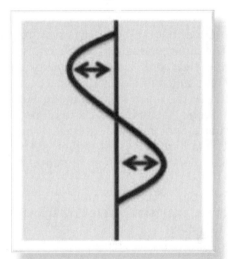

One quantum is a wavelength starting from a centerline, lifting out to a maximum to one side. It then returns past the centerline and extends into the opposite side with exactly the same intensity.

In nature, there is no attribute for the left side being positive and the right being negative. Both sides just are and are interchanging permanently. Every wave is symmetrical on both sides of the centerline, as shown in the diagram.

First Conclusion:

One quantum, which is the smallest building block from which all things are made, contains both a so-called positive and negative charge.

Second Conclusion:

Everything that is built out of many quanta is equally positive and negative.

Example: If you measure a magnet, you will see that it has a positive charge on one end and a negative charge at the other end. If you then break the magnet exactly in half, you will find that you do not have a negative and a positive half, but two pieces which are equally positive and negative.

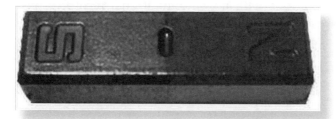

Thus, you cannot remove this positive/negative duality from anything or anyone. Duality will always exist to equal measures.

Emotional Awareness

☯ THE CAUSE OF EMOTION

To understand the concept of emotions, you must first understand where they come from. To do this, you have to check your memory.

Try to remember what you were doing seven years ago on Tuesday, June 23rd. You will not have any particular memory, unless you experienced a significant event on that day. You will only remember that specific date if your spouse left you, a tragic accident occurred, you had your first kiss, your child was born or some kind of memorable event took place.

You will remember only those things, which you judged as either very GOOD or very BAD. The greater the emotional charge, the stronger the memory.

Boring memories with no emotional charge are forgotten. They evaporate into thin air.

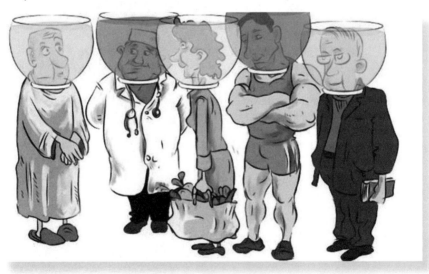

When I see people arguing, imagine that everybody has a bowl filled with their BELIEFS and CHARGES over their head and, based on the content, they see the world completely different. Each one of them is certain to be right and everybody else is wrong.

This is what a patient experiences when he or she is trying to find common ground. No matter whom they ask, they will always get different opinions. The doctor will have opinions he has learned at school to be true. He believes medicine is the solution. The sports teacher might have a completely different belief and rather tries to focus on exercise and detoxification. The green-juice lady will think all others are completely nuts. You need rest and loads of her vegetables to recover.

So who is correct? All of them? None? The truth is that they all see the problem through the filter of their own experiences beliefs.

To find a solution for yourself, you need to find your own truth. There is no short cut and the result will be from what you experience. If you have chemotherapy and get well, then this is your truth. If you have juices and enemas and you get well, then this is your truth. But it's a tinted truth, which only fits to you and no one else.

Imagine all of them to gurgle with bubbles, and no one else can understand what they are trying to convey.

The problem is that no one knows that their viewpoints and beliefs are tinted.

☯ CHARGED MEMORIES DETERMINE YOUR BEHAVIOUR

Before we discuss the effects of emotion, let's look at a few scenarios, which make this whole play very transparent.

As a child, you unconsciously realize that, when sick, your mother spends extra time with you. Her normally very busy schedule is tossed aside, and you are in the limelight with her full attention. You get a lot of extra affection and tender loving care.

This can lead to an unconscious pattern, which can manipulate the body to get sick in order to receive more love. It's an unconscious motivation, which can be lethal.

Your parents gave you sweets to brighten you up as a child when you were down or sad. Guess what you need when you feel bad as an adult?

Perhaps they gave you sweets to celebrate an achievement. Guess what you need when you celebrate success as an adult?

If a bald man in blue jeans beat your mother and you observed the pain it caused when you were little, you would unconsciously restrain from being around bald men dressed in blue jeans. You would unconsciously avoid everyone with no hair, no matter how nice this person might be.

This example shows that any kind of prejudice is truly limiting and you might miss many opportunities, just because of an unconscious judgment.

You can even take up likes and dislikes from authorities like parents and teachers. Without ever experiencing any bad situation yourselves, you take part in judgment based on what you are told. A good example would be casting a political vote based on your parents' opinion. Your religious choice, to which God you should pray, without deciding for yourself what you believe, is another excellent example. These subconscious charges will cause you to be opposed to different religions or races just because you were told to do so.

These emotional memories have a tight grip on you, as they are stored in the subconscious or unconscious mind. You don't even realize how they manipulate you. Unconsciously, you are a victim of your own perceptions.

If you have a problem in any area of life including health, please understand that these are symptoms of the unconscious beliefs from which you operate.

CONCLUSION:

Every charge causes unconscious reactions!

The reaction can range from an embarrassed smile to an intense steaming off all red-faced, or you could even be physically lashing out at the offender. Depending on your emotional charges, the same incident can cause different reactions.

You can observe this when a friend is completely outraged about a comment, which does not even touch you. You wonder why something, which is completely insignificant for you, can cause your friend to over-react.

Every emotion is expressed physically and has an effect on your body. It may be in the form of tummy ulcers, tense shoulders or back pain, but no matter how it manifests, it will cause some kind of physical reaction within the body.

This is why many say that positive emotions like joy, gratitude and laughter have a relaxing and healing influence on the body; whereas stress, fear and frustration have devastating effects on your health.

Health Effects Of Emotions

In ancient times, the wise and knowledgeable Rishis in India studied the effects of emotions. They covered all the emotions and related diseases in the Upanishads and the Jyotishshastras. They created many different tables to show the correlation between emotions and physical expression. These tables are very helpful to find the emotion responsible for disease. In fact, they were used to help a person to heal.

Some of the most obvious ones are:

Grief, depression, hopelessness, sorrow and similar emotional feelings are often related to old age, death and decay. These emotions lead to chronic diseases and constitutional and congenial wasting and weakness. Under this domain are constipation, inability to discharge waste materials, low vitality, poor resistance, and poor absorption of nutrients, which causes numbness, stiffness, rigidity and spasms. These types of emotions lead to arthritis, rheumatism, premature aging, osteoporosis, nervous disorders, paralysis, multiple sclerosis, Parkinson's, and cancer. Grief and hopelessness are also related to deficiencies of vital fluids, dehydration, pain and itch.

Greed, envy, want, obsession, and fear of loss lead to nervous disorders and possession on a psychic level. They cause suicidal tendencies and manic depression, insomnia, bad dreams, palpitations, nervous disorders, insanity and paralysis. If no balance is found, cancer is a common result due to the suppression of the immune system. They cause nervous digestion, loss of appetite and parasites to develop. They are also the cause of hormonal imbalances and all kinds of mysterious pains and diseases.

Suppressed or outspoken anger, fury, resentment, frustration, impatience, stress, impulsiveness and any excessive negative emotion often intensify inner and outer bleeding, the effects of surgery, infections, high fever, absorption of high toxin levels, acute febrile and infectious diseases. In general, these emotions cause fever, inflammation and burning sensations; as well as hypertension. They are mostly responsible for liver and gall bladder disorders including cancer. The most common conditions associated with these emotions are - acne, boils, ulcerative sores, herpes, and venereal diseases. Cancer of the blood, particularly leukemia, is found to be a frequent result of suppressed anger.

Addiction, desire, missing out, never enough emotions are associated with disorders of the kidneys, reproductive organs, and are often the reason for impotency, menstrual irregularity, pain and cramping. A tendency to miscarriages will exist. Chronic kidney and bladder infections are common and even kidney and gall stones. This will often lead to urinary incontinence, swollen prostates, cysts and problems of the skin. There will always be a disorder with hormones and body fluids when these emotions are present.

False optimism or pessimism, lack of self-confidence, bad luck and blame emotions result in overweight, edema, diabetes, poor circulation, weak liver function and heart diseases. Tumors are often associated with these feelings. All kinds of excess organ growth, lack of strength, cough, and shortness of breath, nervous disorders, and hormonal imbalances are a direct result of these emotions.

These relationships are only indications and not the sole cause of the conditions they are associated with. A variety of elements will be present and when these elements are combined, they will play a vital role in causing illness in your body. But the main focus of this lesson is that there is never an emotional reaction without a physical influence on our health.

That's why you need to become conscious of the emotions in the first place and then search for the belief, which drives this emotion.

☯ DISCHARGING YOUR MEMORIES

As you probably have noticed, there are certain things, which make you happy or angry, while other people remain completely untouched by them. The reason for this is that they do not have the same emotional charge as you do. Some people might see what you fear as something pleasant or positive, or they may view something you love as being absolutely stupid or appalling. The only difference is the emotional charge and the belief you hold in your subconscious mind.

The first step in healing the body through the mind is by discharging the belief, which drives the emotion.

The tool to discharge your emotions is a UNIVERSAL LAW, which is called:

Everything has equal and complementary opposites.

Up/down, full/empty, day/night, light/dark, front/back, top/bottom, ugly/pretty, good/bad and so on. Nothing comes without a complementary opposite. And both sides are always present at exactly the same time. You will never have one without the other. You may see only one side at a time, but you know the other is there. Take day and night as an example. Once it's night, you may not see the sunshine, but nevertheless you know it's there. If you could move up into space, you would be able to see both.

This LAW can be found in every situation of life. Once you know what to look for, you will see it immediately.

Have you ever wondered why, anywhere in the world, people can't agree on the same outcome when discussing a problem?

Why doesn't everybody like caviar? Why do some say oysters are the best things on earth, while others gag when they have to eat them?

Have you ever tried to eat the Swiss specialty, which they call stinkerkaess? It's a cheese which smells so bad you could faint. Upon unwrapping you want to rip all windows open to be able to breathe. It's disgusting, but they love it. They sit with glassy eyes and enjoy the smell and the taste.

There are hundreds of examples when you speak about food and specialties in particular, but you could also look at simple things like ice cream. I think we all agree that ice cream is all-good. It is delicious. But is it really? When you look into the list of ingredients, you might reconsider your judgment. Especially when you list all the stabilizers, flavors, colors, food enhancers, preservatives and artificial flavors. And even if it's a healthy all-organic ice cream (which usually does not taste as good), it kills your digestive fire, gives you an energy breakdown and lowers your immune response. The sugar in the icecream makes you hyper and destroys your teeth. Plus it is addicting and costs money, which means you need to work longer and harder to afford this so-called luxury. Then think of the chain reaction. If you have one, the whole family wants one as well. Which is even more expensive. And just to mention it, there are many people who would not eat icecream. They think it's disgusting. Hard to believe, but I know a few who would never touch it due to the sugar overload.

There is an opposition to every political party, religions fight with each other, there is peace and war at all times around the world and, even though it's right in our face all the time, NO ONE wants to realize that there is no good without bad.

All of mankind strives to achieve the impossible. And no matter how obvious it is, they never give up.

CONCLUSION

Everything is good and bad at the same time. In fact, everything is NEUTRAL. It's only the perception of the observer, which gives it the charge.

Here are a few examples, which describe the same thing as good and bad:

GOOD: A doctor, for example, views DISEASE as a good thing. The more people who are sick, the better, because that's how they earn money. Cancer is a multi-million dollar business, so is heart disease and everything else. There are hundreds of professionals and institutions benefiting from our health-related issues and they call disease a good thing; without it, they would be out-of-business.

BAD: But if you look more carefully, there are plenty of drawbacks as well if people are sick. Doctors are statistically under a great deal of stress. They must deal with angry and frustrated patients and relatives. They work long hours. When they realize they cannot help their patient, depression and suicidal tendencies are common. Higher authorities (pharmaceuticals) tell them what to do, legal obligations, book keeping, staff problems, and many more are factors that exist in their daily lives. Not to mention all of the antibiotic resistant bugs and related diseases they have to deal with while being in a hospital.

GOOD: Even the purpose of a doctor has many different angles. On the one hand, they are good for treatment of injuries, broken bones, sprains, cuts and bruises.

BAD: But, on the other hand, their method of treating degenerative disease is unproductive, and the medications they use have more side effects than they help.

BAD: From a patient's point of view, is DISEASE always a bad thing? Well, it is often accompanied by pain, it's expensive and it takes a lot of effort to get well. Disease is known to stop you in your tracks; making it difficult, if not impossible, to continue on the same path as you were before. It also causes a lot of fear and requires you to make changes in your lifestyle, which is probably the greatest drawback of all.

GOOD: But then again, patients report benefits from being sick. They don't have to go to work or they can escape their daily routine. Some welcome the act of being taken care of by someone else. Others might use it as a testament and get involved in speaking about their illness; it gives them something worthwhile to do and becomes their passion. For many elderly patients, it's actually a highlight of the week to have a doctor's appointment. The social aspect involved in sharing their condition with someone who is looking after them is something they often look forward to. The disease forces many patients to bring their affairs in order. And many finally learn to look after their body. They learn about nutrition, detoxification, exercise and joy and laughter. Many of the patients we have talked to say that cancer was the greatest blessing in their life.

Depending on your primary focus, you can look at the same thing from many different angles and judge it to be good or bad or both.

True healing of the mind does not come from chasing after the so-called good side until you get it. It comes from the realization that, in essence, everything is NEUTRAL.

When I first realized this simple law, I developed in 2005 a workshop, which was called "Loving Cancer." At first, I was kind of ridiculed, but soon this changed due to the feedback and the results we achieved. The course was designed to guide a patient to find the blessings, since they were diagnosed with cancer. Due to our inherent nature of judging things single-sided, most patients had a hard time to make the connections, but with a bit of practice this changed and all of them could find a minimum of 100 and often up to 250 blessings in disguise.

We call these blessings **"GIFTS IN SHITTY WRAPPING PAPER,"** as instigated by the famous actor Tony Barry. And that's what they are.

These blessings are there for everybody. The problem is that most people don't connect them with the cause and do not acknowledge them as such, but nevertheless they are there.

I have to admit sometimes it's really hard to believe in this law and in some cases even I come to doubt that there is anything good to find. But every single time I am shown again that nothing happens by chance. I have led clients through this exercise who have lost a loved one, who went bankrupt, had an ugly divorce, who were abused or beaten, or had lost their house in a flood without insurance, and every single time we can find the blessings unfold in mysterious ways.

The biggest problem is that you cannot hypothetically find blessings. You have to experience it. You can only find the blessings when you go through this ordeal.

This process is partly very simple and easy. You just need to start looking with open eyes and slowly take off the filter, through which you see the world. The hard part is, wanting to let go of your addiction to blame. It's so convenient to blame others for your misery. Seeing the perfection in everything, that happens, requires courage.

Let me tell you a real-case scenario, which was actually my introduction to cancer:

During my early years in Australia, I was offering a coaching service for individuals who searched the blessings in shitty wrapping paper. I was very well booked from all walks of life. Then, one day, a young lady called. She was probably in her mid-40s. She booked an appointment, telling me she wanted to know the purpose of her life. As this was my main passion at the time, I agreed and we booked a time the very next day due to her urgency. When she came, I was shocked to see that she was in her final stages of a very serious disease. She had to be carried to my office and was very weak.

After a short introduction, Ulrike started to laugh and asked me to relax. She said, "It's me who is dying not you. So relax," which in a way broke the ice. At that time, I had never been confronted with a person so close to death. At least not visibly, which made me feel kind of insecure.

As I had described before it is not always easy at first glance to see the blessings, especially in a case like that where all seems lost, but after my initial panic of not being able to deliver, we started the process which I had done so many times and I asked her to tell me everything that had transformed to the good since she was diagnosed with cancer in her case.

Her outburst of outrage was imminent. She immediately tried to convince me that there was nothing good. "Just look at me and then ask the same question again," she almost yelled at me. As I was used to this kind of reaction, I just kept asking the same question again and again with slight hints of suggestions.

For example, I changed my question to, "What has changed to the good in regards to your spiritual life, since you have been diagnosed with cancer?" "Have you learned or discovered or read something which you could call an improvement?"

That's when she started to see the connection and just alone in the department of spirituality we found about 25 changes to the positive.

Books she read and loved.

Friends she made at meditation groups.

One particular friend who had actually brought her to me.

The Tibetan Book of the Living and Dying was a huge influence and support.

Her anger against dogmatic forms of religion had turned into an understanding of the needs which drove this form of belief.

Her own spiritual journey had begun with hopelessness and opened a lot of doors and insights.

She has also had personal experiences during meditation, which convinced her of a life after death.

And many more.

- Once she was on a roll, it was very easy to move on to the next theme. It's as if the mind needs a training to see connections. Usually, the good and the bad are separate and have nothing to do with each other. But that's not so.

- The next subject proved to be the winner, as I looked for subjects that might be the main contributors to her disease. I asked her what had changed in the relationship with her parents since she was diagnosed with cancer. After a little hesitation, she then told me a story which was tear-jerking. She had a fall out with her mother about 14 years ago and had not spoken to either her dad or mum for that time. She also had refused all contact with her sister who was then the culprit for the argument and her leaving home.

- After the diagnoses, she all of a sudden had this huge urge and desire to see her family. It was a thought she could not delete from her mind. After standing at the corner to the house for several days, she finally overcame her fear of rejection and knocked at the door. She was extremely anxious that her parents would not want her anymore after how she had behaved, but when the door opened and her mum saw her, she burst into tears, hugged her in a tight embrace and pulled her into the house.

- This hug was the biggest relief she had ever experienced. This whole process of kissing, hugging and embracing continued with her dad who was suffering from Alzheimer's. Even though most of the time he did not remember who his wife was, he remembered his daughter and did not let her go.

- Well, at this point of her realization, we all joined in with our tears. It was an overwhelming moment of realization where she could see the perfect order of the universe.

- I will spare you the rest as relationship did go on forever. It was the culprit for her disease and, only after realizing that cancer had helped her mend at least half of her relationships, she had found the purpose of cancer in her life.

- In this process, we go through all the seven areas of life and ask the same question in many different forms and to different subjects in order to trigger their mind to see the higher order.
- After our session, which went very long, Ulrike started to process all the things which were still OPEN / CHARGED. It was a beautiful process and we became very good friends.

CONCLUSION

The most obvious conclusion you can draw from the above is that you have to be grateful for the gifts in shitty wrapping paper. They help you solve what the psyche could not solve on its own.

The second conclusion you can draw from this experience is that no one but YOU is in charge of how you perceive this world.

If you see everything as bad and scary and you have set beliefs which support your judgment, it's not because a person or thing or relationship is bad, but because you see only the negative side.

If you see everything as good and wonderful and you have big illusions, it's not because a person or thing is good, but because you see only the positive side.

☯ EVERYONE HAS TWO SIDES

Sometimes it's quite logical to see that items and things are neutral in essence and only your emotional charges make them positive or negative. However, in the case of enemies and idols, it's much harder to see and certainly to admit. We are so attached to a single-sided illusion that we do not want to see this universal law in action.

Let's look, for example, at Mother Theresa. In all of our workshops, someone always mentions her name when I ask for a person who has no drawbacks, no criticism, no blame, no enemies; someone who is ALL GOOD. Everybody loves her.

But is this so?

Well, I know a lot of families who are very upset with her because they tried to adopt a child and did not fit into the religious dogma that was required.

Others were very upset to find that the millions of dollars she received in donations were not used for the kids and poor as intended, but were handed over to the Vatican. Instead, she invested the money she received into missionary work to convert all of the lost Hindus into Christians. In India, when you ask about Mother Theresa, you hear very few kind words because of that.

Many were outright shocked to see that all the babies under Mother Theresa's care could not even sit or stand at the age of 3 because they were never taken out of their beds. These babies had serious developmental problems due to a lack of attention from the few volunteers and nuns who were ordered to help.

I have personally visited the orphanages in Delhi, Calcutta and Mumbai and each time I was more frustrated than the time before to see the desperation of helpers who tried to help, but were not allowed to do so. Everything was kept to a bare minimum, despite the millions of donations.

When we asked Mother Theresa why she did not allow toys and more playtimes, she said that she did not want to interfere with the children's karma; they were born into poverty and had to remain there. The suffering of Christ was their destiny. Hitchens described Mother Teresa's organization as a cult, which promoted suffering. And indeed, this is what she caused.

There were many investigations against Mother Theresa due to her financial dealings and her involvement in politics.

She was also involved in an unpopular population control campaign, which involved forcible sterilization, resulting in huge criticism and a strong lobby against her.

When I began to research Mother Teresa, I actually felt myself very disillusioned, as there are a lot more negative aspects to consider. I don't want to be the one who bursts your bubble, so I will allow you to conduct your own research; but even Mother Theresa has equal complementary opposites.

In all fairness, we have actually conducted this same exercise on many other publicly prominent people and there is no single-sided outcome. There is always both. Take Michael Jackson or Lady Gaga, they have or had millions of fans, while millions don't like them at all! Study the life of the Dalai Lama and the Pope and you will find plenty of support and challenge in their life. If you prefer to go into politics, look at President Obama and George W. Bush; they are living proof that everyone has two sides.

You can also look at religions and organizations. The same law is at work there.

As a less prominent person, I thought to share my own experiences by creating my DVD "CANCER Is Curable NOW" and the Workbook to the movie. If I had hoped for a single-sided praise and glory without any criticism, I would now probably sit in a corner and cry.

I have received plenty of criticism. Not only from conventional doctors, but even some holistic doctors do not approve of my work. Some feel threatened by our compilation and say it's giving too many choices. Others thought I had missed their particular miracle cure and said I had offered too few choices. Then there are people who think that the DVD and Book should be free. They think it should be for the common good of mankind and I am a greedy, profit-hungry person to charge for my years of work and research. Others say I should charge more for it. There are even whole groups of people who call me a charlatan who is leading people into certain death. And there are those who feel I am bashing the conventional doctors too much, and so on.

Plus there are certainly those who love what we are doing and support us.

It all depends on what kind of a program is stored in a person's subconscious mind. (Fishbowl over their head!!!) If they believe all people should be converted to Christianity, they will support Mother Theresa and think she did the right thing. If they gave money to help the kids and then saw it was used for missionary work, then they think it's bad.

But in truth everything and everyone just is. Nothing is either good or bad. It's both. Mother Theresa was not evil, nor was she a saint. She was a human being with emotional charges, which motivated her to do what she did. And so am I and everybody else. We all live by our emotional charges and, by doing so, try to resolve them.

We will discuss what this means in the following chapters.

CONCLUSION:

In the early stages of this chapter, I just want you to become aware of complementary opposites. They are everywhere and you just need to look for them.

If you regard something as positive, search for the negative and become aware of the balance. Find people who dislike what you like and check their arguments. They have a different fishbowl over their head and therefore see things differently.

If you regard something as negative, search for all the benefits, opportunities, blessings, lessons, learning experiences, opposite opinions and become aware of the balance.

If you feel supported, find the challenge. (It's there at the same time.)

If you feel challenged, find the support. (It's there at the same time.) This particular exercise is easy to observe in a family. For example: Father yelling, "Joseph, eat your broccoli. You won't get off the tale until you've done so! Joseph starts crying. Mother to father, "Don't yell at my darling. Now you've frightened him."

With four kids and a wife, I could tell you 200 of these support and challenge stories. And even if parents are not involved, there is always a friend, grandparent or a neighbor who joins the club of emotional exchange.

If you feel admired, find those who think you are horrible. (No need to cheat. We know they are there. It's by law!)

If someone steals from you, look for those who are giving.

If someone praises you, look for those who are criticizing AT THE SAME TIME!

Everything is in perfect balance, all the time. You just need to become aware of it.

Friends, supporters, fans, followers	Enemies, critics, challengers, opposition

Sometimes, one person hates you so much that they can compensate for a few who just like you. That's why you don't count people, but volume of emotion.

☯ EVIDENCE DOES NOT MAKE SOMETHING TRUE

An emotionally charged viewpoint is always lopsided. Therefore, you have to prove to yourself and others, that you are right. It's like a curse.

For instance, if you think "all men are untruthful," you will constantly be looking for evidence to prove your charge. You will find friends who agree with your viewpoint and see the same problem in their relationships. You will also find evidence in movies, songs and the news reports. Sometimes, you even create situations to prove to yourself that you are right.

If you think that all conventional doctors are bad and only kill people with their chemotherapy, you will also try to convince yourself and others of your lopsided beliefs. You will find articles and magazines, which support your claim. You will have ears like a radar dish to hear whatever supports your claims.

Unfortunately, all of this evidence does not make this lopsided viewpoint correct and many will challenge you. You can find just as much evidence for "all men are truthful" or "all doctors are helpful and caring" if you look for it

In reality, they are both. In matters of importance, men are truthful and if they try to cheat their way out, they are untruthful. Doctors are caring and at the same time don't hesitate to use what's common practice.

Every charged emotion will cause you to collect evidence to prove your point.

A doctor we met on our journey claimed that cancer was caused by inflammations and, no matter how many patients he treated, he found inflammation as the main cause. He had gathered hundreds of papers and evidence to support his case, and if you look at his documentation, he was correct in many ways. When we asked him how he came to this conclusion, he explained that his wife had passed away after battling cancer for many years. Her main problems were inflammations in the joints, Candida and intestinal inflammations which suppressed the immune system.

One doctor was convinced that all cancer was caused by emotional trauma and every patient he treated confirmed his theory. He had documented over 4,080 cases to prove his point. His emotional charge, which had been the cause for his research, was his own cancer four years after his son had been killed. He was convinced that every cancer is related to emotional trauma.

Another doctor was convinced that toxins caused cancer, another by deficiencies and the next was convinced he had found the cause to be a virus, and his evidence was overwhelming too. He had hundreds of documents showing that HE was right.

All of them are correct and incorrect at the same time. What they have observed is only one side of the truth as instigated by their charge.

Many things cause cancer and the combination of factors is only going to increase the risk. There might be inflammations together with deficiencies, or emotional trauma combined with toxins. Combine all four contributing factors and you are nearing the truth.

CONCLUSION

Every lopsided observation requires proof to others and to yourself. If you feel compelled to defend your viewpoint, you should look at your judgment and consider the belief, which drives it. There is a lopsided / single-sided / charged memory in your subconscious mind which determines your behavior. This charge has control over you.

Dissolve it and you are free.

☯ EMOTIONAL CHARGES DETERMINE YOUR SUCCESS AND FAILURE

Based on your emotional charges, you will have likes and dislikes.

Positive charges lead to empowered areas of life, because you are drawn to them, spend time with them and invest energy to learn more.

Negative charges lead to disempowered areas of life, because you avoid and neglect them.

These likes and dislikes lead to a hierarchy of values.

If you invest plenty of time and passion into finances, for example, you will learn how to handle money wisely. You will gain experience and, over time, manage to make money work for you.

You will also become a master of HEALTH if you invest time, money and energy into the study and maintenance of the human body. With practice, you will learn to listen to your own physical reactions and know what's good for you and what's not.

Many lessons need to be learned to get you from a disempowered state to a mastery in all areas of life, and you will only go through all these difficulties if your emotionally charged memories in your subconscious mind allow you to do so.

Strong dislikes, aversions, judgments, negative memories, resentment, polarized opinions and bad experiences will certainly hold you back or cause you to deviate from your plans.

That's why, no matter how often you start, you will always fail to achieve your goals if you do not discharge your negative beliefs.

Charged memories can be compared with a software program.

Negative charge = walk away / don't do / ignore / run / avoid

Positive charge = get more / do now / want / appreciate / enjoy

If you want to see how you are programmed, you only need to look at your life. It will reflect clearly what areas of life are programmed with negative charges and which ones are supported with positive charges.

☯ THE SEVEN AREAS OF LIFE

FINANCIAL

Positive charges will create a lot of money and you have it working for you. Financial power is always expressed if you know how to create and maintain wealth.

Negative financial charges are indicators that you owe money, don't have enough money, can't repay and can't afford. Money runs through your fingers like water and you can't save it.

RELATIONSHIPS

Positive charges will create great relationships with your loved ones. If you support your partner in their passion for life and they do the same for you. If you are able to really communicate with your partner and understand each other.

Negative charges show in your RELATIONSHIPS when you feel alone. If you have no one to share your life with and no one who cares for you or no one to care for. Disempowerment in this area also leads to envy, anger, meanness, dishonesty, resentment and stress.

SOCIAL

Positive charges will create authority. People listen to your advice, accept you as a leader and you have authority in your field. You will have plenty of fans and enemies when you are socially empowered.

Negative charges show if your SOCIAL actions are not accepted by society and no one follows your lead.

PHYSICAL

Positive charges will result in a healthy and well-trained body and the knowledge to maintain health in an educated way.

Negative charges show when your body is experiencing disease and a weak physical condition. Especially if you have no knowledge on how to help yourself.

MENTAL

Positive charges will be evident when you have degrees and expertise in your field of passion. If you are able to share what you have learned and others accept you as the one who knows.

Negative MENTAL charges show when you exhibit problems with concentration, have difficulty memorizing and no ability or desire to learn. Your level of education is low and your verbal and mental expressions are limited.

VOCATIONAL

Positive charges will be expressed in a top-level career in whatever you do. You love what you do and do what you love. You have a thriving business or employment.

Negative VOCATIONAL charges show when there is little success in your career, if you hate what you do and do what you hate. If your career does not take you towards your goals but keeps you under constant pressure.

SPIRITUAL

Positive charges will be expressed in knowing your life purpose and knowing why you are here on earth. They give you the certainty and motivation to move forward with life.

Negative VOCATIONAL charges show when you are not motivated, lack passion, frequently change directions, practice trial and error with no satisfaction and aimlessly wander from one promise of happiness to the next.

EXERCISE 4

For the next short exercise, I would like you to first find your own hierarchy of values.

What does your life demonstrate? Where do you have the most success? Which area of your life is thriving? Where do you have the most positive charges?

As you continue building this list, you will reach those areas of life, which are not as empowered and, typically, cause a lot of stress. These are the areas of life, which are negatively charged.

Write your most successful area into the first box (1). Write your most troubled, stressed and negatively charged area in the last box (7). All others have to be sorted in between.

Set them into the perfect hierarchy as your life demonstrates.

Areas of life are:

Spiritual, Relational, Physical, Mental, Financial, Social and Career

You	Your Spouse / Partner / Parent / Enemy Name:
1.)	
2.)	
3.)	
4.)	
5.)	
6.)	
7.)	

The second column is where you can list the person whom you feel challenged by in that area. It might be your partner, parent, employer, co-worker, enemy or friend.

Note their hierarchy of values compared to yours. Those areas, which are at the opposite ends, will have highly opposing charges and therefore cause you to have stress, fights and arguments.

☯ DIFFERENT VALUES CAUSE FIGHTS

No matter how hard you try, you won't be able to make it good for everybody. A mother will know this very well. No matter how good her intentions are, someone will always be upset and of a different opinion.

As long as people support your emotional charges and values and agree with you, you call them friends. You like to be with them and describe them as nice, charming, interesting, good and pleasant to be around. But as soon as someone challenges your values/viewpoints, you don't like them and you try to avoid them, especially if they are strongly opposed in their own opinion.

So don't think that your friends love you no matter what. They are only your friends as long as you support their values.

A conflict will usually occur if someone with low values connects with someone with high values in the same field. As both parties are very passionate in extreme polar opposites, the clash is unavoidable.

This can be seen with sports fanatics. If you share the interest and participate in the discussion, you are cool. If you are brave enough to say you hate soccer, you are not so cool. Usually, such a comment leads to exclusion from the group. You criticize what they love.

If you place a great value on HEALTH and you have developed and educated yourself in this field through painful experience and research, you will try to influence your family and friends to follow your lead. If they do, you are happy.

But if your son or daughter or wife smokes or enjoys junk food and fills the fridge with GMO, Aspartame, MSG and all other poisons, you will be challenged. They will drive you mad.

On the opposite side, your family may call you paranoid and over the top and may be frustrated with your nagging.

Values separate us or unite us.

SOLUTION:

Do you remember the law of equal complementary opposites? That every extreme emotional charge has, by law, a complementary opposite?

This also applies in clashing values.

If you are a health fanatic, you will attract or be attracted to those who do not care about health at all. Their job is to balance you out. The more you try to enforce a diet of all organic, raw, healthy foods, the more they buy GMO, MSG and Aspartame-laden, dead foods, which are filled with artificial flavors and colors.

If you observe your own family dynamics, you will find this LAW of **equal complementary opposites** everywhere and it fits into every area of life.

- A person who places a high value on being wealthy will always have a family member or friend who prefers to spend their money and has no interest in holding on to it.
- A person who has an incredible thirst for knowledge and studies the most advanced literature will have a partner who watches soap operas and reads junk magazines.
- A person who is obsessively tidy will have a messy partner who keeps messing up the house.
- A person who has a high value in social recognition will have a controversial partner who does not care what others think.

This partner can be a spouse, child, parent, family member or friend.

So what do you think you must learn in order to escape these oppositions? What is the universe trying to tell you?

Could it be that you are forced to become aware of your own emotional charges so that you can discharge them?

- Fanatic charges / beliefs cause fights, violence, protests and war.
- Strong charges / beliefs cause strong arguments and separation.
- Little charges / beliefs cause little arguments.
- No charges / beliefs will bring peace and harmony.

In my childhood and increasingly during my teens, I experienced extreme stress caused by the dress code of our family. My mother was obsessively concerned that we were dressed properly, hair all tidy and according to the situation. My dad never wore anything else than suit and tie, and my sister owned one of the most exclusive and prestigious designer boutiques in our town. Pullovers cost up to $2,000 each. And I had to wear them to fit the picture. Guess what I had to balance out as soon as I had outgrown the moaning and complaining state. I was the hippy of the family. Spiritual outfit and ripped jeans made for the daily clash. From teens on, this intensified into a war, which in the end drove me to the other side of the world into the outskirts of Puri in India, just to escape. This was, as it turned out, **my gift in shitty wrapping paper**, as I learned so much and got to know my Jyotish community and my teachers that I am happy today for the drama I had at home.

Instead of escaping, there would have been a much more emotionally intelligent approach. Accepting my family's desire to dress well and appreciate their values by recognizing the success they have and how well they look.

If I wanted something really bad and needed support, I could gain their trust by fitting into their values.

If I wanted an excuse and escape, I could go opposite and the clash was programmed.

This would have been the salesman / businessman approach. Appreciate the values of your clients and fit in so that they trust and support you.

For myself, without the salesman attitude, I could still dress according to my own values in my own and private time and if I want their acceptance, dress according to their values without negating my own deepest values. Organic cotton and non-toxic clothing was mandatory.

This would be the peaceful approach where I do not try to change others. This is in essence what it boils down to. Trying to convince and change others to what I believe to be the best. Trying to pour some of my tinted water into their fishbowls over their heads.

Emotional unintelligent people try to convince and, if that does not work, fight, oppose and defend their beliefs.

Emotionally intelligent people appreciate other people's values, but do not negate their own.

You can still do what you like and eat as much organic food as you want, as long as you do not try to force it onto others. You can still choose to pray to your god, but you do not need to convert others to the same belief. You can still dress in designer clothes, but you don't need to criticize others if they don't.

In the same way, you don't need to be upset if someone criticizes you; just smile and become aware of their beliefs emotional charges and motivations. Don't be offended, they just lack the emotional intelligence to love you the way you are. Therefore, they try to transform you into what they think is better (based on their values).

Imagine a meadow full of flowers. If one flower thought she was the most beautiful flower in the meadow and wanted all the flowers to change their appearance to be just like her, how ignorant would that be?

If you really want to change your world around you, inspire them. Be the change you want to see in this world. If you radiate what you try to change and it appeals to others, some will follow on their own accord.

How is that for a thought?

One of my coaching clients, James Laurell shared a story with me which is really to the point:-

> *Once upon a time, I was one of those radical, judgmental and emotional vegetarians and only associated with people who shared my beliefs. In fact, for many years, I was quite a challenge for many of my fellow humans as I made it my passion to point out the horrible conditions of conventionally grown meats. I posted videos of animal slaughter and transport conditions and short movies, which pointed out the injustice and hygiene conditions.*

It was a fanatic position which took up a lot
of my mental space and my emotions were
at the mercy of my surroundings. I did not
even like to eat in places where they cooked
meat. Just the thought of it disgusted me.

Well, guess what kind of opposition I attracted.
Besides the continuous ridicule of friends,
my father was my biggest challenger. He
prepared a huge roast, or any other animal,
each time we came to visit and only served a
tiny portion of vegetables. Preferably, he used
the meat sauce to season the veggies. Or he
used chicken broth to make us a vegetarian
soup. When we did not watch out carefully, he
fed supermarket sausages to my kids and told
them not to say anything to me. My father-
in-law, brothers-in-law, as well as some of
my friends, challenged me in similar ways.
Then, one day, inspired by Marcus and his
teachings I decided to discharge my opinions
and beliefs over meat and searched for over 50
benefits of eating meat. Guess what? It was not
hard at all, and some points were even very
convincing. I also searched for 50 drawbacks
in being a vegetarian, and found these very
easily. Social harassment was certainly on the
top of the list, but there were also some serious
health-related discoveries, which helped to
tip the scale. Already, during the process of
discharge, I felt so much lighter and more
peaceful than before. The following week, I
bought some organic, grass-fed meat and
ate it secretly with my wife to check out if we
would die on the spot. It was actually delicious
and we now have a small portion once or twice
a month with our children who are really
excited. I can't say that I need it, but it does no
harm either. On the contrary, I feel very good.

> *The biggest and most relaxing factor though,*
> *was to drop this extreme charge which was*
> *certainly unhealthier than eating factory*
> *farmed meat from the supermarket.*

No matter what your charge is, you will always have the same amount of support and challenge.

I think it's very obvious from the example above, that, whatever charge and value you have, you will have an opposition. Some will think you are great and chime in with their support, and others feel challenged or criticized and will oppose your view.

Once you change your viewpoint, you will see that the support and challenge just flip like a flag in the wind. Those who supported vegetarianism were now against James and all meat eaters applauded. The result is still the same.

Which means...

No matter what you do, you will always have friends and enemies. You will always have support and challenge. If your viewpoints are extreme, you will attract extreme opposition as well as support. If you have a little charge, you will have little opposition. But if you have no charge, you will have peace.

As a little exercise, you can observe your own family. Who has an extreme charge? Who is the supporter and who challenges? You will always have this configuration at work.

CONCLUSION

Relax and let others be how they want to be. As soon as you drop your charges, life is much less challenging.

Follow your dreams and do what you think you have to do. Some will like it and others will hate you for it. No matter how hard you try, you won't have everybody on your side.

Once I got this, and I mean once it clicked in my head, I felt as if 100 tons of weight were taken of my shoulders. The constant struggle to be good and all perfect so that **everybody** loves and admires me was a huge stress. Especially since you never reach this illusion.

☯ VOIDS DRIVE VALUES / UNWANTED MOTIVATION

Now let's look at one of the universal, self-regulating laws, which are a blessing in disguise.

"VOIDS DRIVE VALUES"

This law wants you to be empowered in all areas of life and, if you aren't it will deprive you of all the pleasures you might find in all other areas of life.

If you dislike a particular area of life, due to negative charged memories, this area will cause problems and eventually infect all other areas of life and spoil the fun.

If you don't learn how to handle your finances, for example, you will be broke. And if you are, every other area of life will suffer. You won't have the money for education, nor for your health. You can't pay your rent and your entire family will suffer. Every other joy is reduced by your inability to handle money.

The same law governs all other areas of life.

Poor health will drag everything down with it. Work, finances, family life, education and so on are all compromised. Pain will spoil everything. If your actions are limited by disease, there is a constant shadow over whatever you do. The effect of medication and the side effects will have a big influence, and toxins, which are produced by many diseases, are clouding your mental capacity. In short, being sick is a huge pain.

When you do not have a job or career, you are unfulfilled and lack a means of support. Relationships usually suffer greatly from a lack of employment. Not to mention the self-worth, which is certainly minimized. No income, no satisfaction, no recognition. Everything is diminished if you have no job.

Luckily, we have this law, which turns whatever you lack most into the most important thing in the world.

If you have no money, for example, you want money more than anything else. Not because money suddenly became important to you and you want a big bank account, but because you want to be able to fulfill your highest values. If you love your family, you need money to send your kids to school or buy a new dishwasher. If your health is important, you need money to buy vitamins and supplements. You need money to join a fitness club and purchase sport equipment and so on.

The Law "Voids Drive Values" is meant to motivate you to evolve, learn, become more and be more. Its purpose is to remind you that you are magnificent and that you can achieve everything.

Life is a journey of growth, adaptation and evolution, and you are not meant to stay behind.

We will cover many more examples later to show you how this law is designed to motivate you to resolve your negative charges. "Voids drive values" is your constant companion, so you'd better get used to the nagging and pushing and follow command. This law will not vanish and leave you in peace. It's your gift in shitty wrapping paper.

In a very extensive study with 20 of my students, we found out that every single person who had achieved remarkable things in this world was motivated by this law.

Think of Mahatma Gandhi. His void was liberty. He had such a strong desire to be independent that he was able to motivate a whole nation to follow.

Think of Mother Theresa. Her void was protection and relief from suffering and through that built an empire.

Many of the doctors we have met were pushed into the study and research about cancer because family members suffered or they had cancer themselves.

CONCLUSION

Be grateful for the VOIDS in your life, they force you to evolve. If these voids didn't require you to improve, you would get used to misery and remain there.

Exercise:

Try to determine the void, which motivates the people around you. I, for instance, see education lacking, as people are manipulated but not educated. So what do I do? I educate research and through that build my little empire.

Your health practitioners might have health problems themselves and try to solve them by helping others. Most psychologists and psychiatrists fall into this category. ☺

If your mother thinks the house is not good enough, her void will drive her to decorate with mountains of deco.

Just become aware of the void and you will see the motivation which drives it.

A good friend of mine from my time in Munich, Bavaria, was very ugly. In fact, she was outstandingly ugly. Her whole face was twisted and out of proportion. Her greatest void was beauty. Guess what she achieved! She was the best interior designer we had in university and her achievements were outstanding. Once on the market, she excelled so fast and was booked out for months with horrendous fees. Her void brought her huge success.

As the exercise, I would like you to look at Steve Jobs and find his void that helped him become one of the greatest contributors in our age. His inventions and ideas have shaped the world and there must be a reason behind this. Write what you find into the comment box in our online version of the book and enlighten us.

This is by far one of the most interesting cases you will find.

Gratitude And love

A great way to heal is when you start to count your blessings and you don't stop until you are overwhelmed by gratitude and love. A clear sign of this overwhelming is when you have tears in your eyes or when your mind chatter resigns and you are completely still and at PEACE. At that moment, you are one with the universe and not battling your beliefs.

In our course, "Loving Cancer," participants reached this point many times and immediately saw improvements in their immune response, healing expedited and the relaxation brought huge benefits into their life. Plus all of them immediately changed their perspective and from then on had a different outlook on life.

A common misunderstanding in this exercise is that most people start listing all of their possessions and good things they have, but is this really what you should be grateful for?

Did any of these luxuries bring you further on your journey of evolution? Did any of these gadgets and possessions make you happy?

We will come back to this, but let's first look at love.

☯   WHAT IS LOVE?

The concept of LOVE has been warped and distorted for generations.

We think we love, if we see the good in others, when we tell them what they want to hear or give them what they want.

We think we are loved when someone tells us what we want to hear and when they give and do what we want.

But, in reality, love is quite a bit more challenging.

Have you realized that when you don't know someone you are polite and mind your own business? But if you get close, you think you have the right to tell your loved ones what you think?

Well, this is often the downfall of many relationships. Especially if you think love is all about pink and sweet. When you first fall in love, you see the world through rose-colored glasses. But once the relationship fades into a daily routine, you feel tempted to speak up and tell them the things you don't like. Likewise, your partner feels the same way. This can make things very turbulent and challenging.

The reason is two-fold:

ONE: Once you get closer, you learn about the weaknesses of your partner. All of a sudden, they are not perfect anymore. You realize their low values in life, and the beliefs which drive their drama. As you become aware of their emotional charges, you get annoyed that they won't get a grip on those issues. At this stage, you start the process of engaging for their greater good. You want to change them, which usually does not work.

TWO: As soon as you enter an emotional relationship, you become the natural balance for your partner. If they get really ambitious and build dream castles, you have to be super realistic. If they are self-minimized, you become the dictator. If they can't decide, you decide for them. If they try to be extra funny, you become extremely serious. If they cheat and lie, you have to be totally honest. If they pray and believe in a god in the clouds, you turn against religion. If they fall on their knees and crawl to touch the feet of the guru, you ridicule them and oppose their behavior. If they drink, you must remain sober. If they are messy, you have to be very orderly.

Whatever stirs your emotions will cause you to equilibrate your relationship.

It's sometimes hard to see, but this balancing act is as much "LOVE" as all the fuzzy, warm and happy feelings. Who else would take this burden upon themselves and balance you out? No one. Who would play the mirror for you if not out of love?

No one else would bother, they would just walk away. We challenge each other out of love so that we evolve. We balance each other, out of love.

> *"There is nothing but love.*
> *All else is an illusion!"*
>
> *- Dr. John F. Demartini*

Do you remember the banker who asks you for money to pay back the mortgage? How he threatened to take your car and house? Well, many would say he was nasty, arrogant and a pain in the butt. But was he really?

If you look at what he did, it's actually the contrary. He pushed you into gear and helped you to empower this area of life. And if you have not mastered it, well then he is probably still pushing. And he won't give up until you make it.

You could even say, "My banker loves me so much that he forces me to get a grip on my finances."

Neale Donald Walsch calls these people who cause us pain in order to motivate us, BLESSINGS in DISGUISE. Read *The Little Soul and the Sun* by Neale and you will fall in love with this concept. It's a lovely story and clearly shows that there are no enemies, but only loving souls who help us to evolve.

Do you remember the doctor who told you that you would die in six months? The one who strongly suggested that you have surgery and chemotherapy immediately, which would completely destroy the last few months of your life?

Do you think he was a BLESSING in DISGUISE?

I assume, if you are reading this book, he actually shocked you into gear. He caused you to focus on your health and learn what's necessary to empower this area of your life. His prognosis was so devastating that you had no other choice but to empower yourself.

Are you grateful that he gave you the death sentence? You should be!

☯ THERE IS NOTHING BUT LOVE!

If you give your child candy **because you love it**, you may cause dental problems, possibly diabetes, all sorts of hyper-activity, reduce their intellect and cause many other health issues.

If you deny your child sweets **because you love it**, they might feel cheated and neglected. They have emotional stress and resentment and think you do not love them.

Whatever you do is the best you can at any given time. Your emotional charge and your beliefs dictate your behavior. You do not have a choice. Whatever is stored in your fishbowl will determine your actions and reactions.

First you will have to have the experience, in order to know what the outcome will be. Once you have learned your lesson, you can decide differently. It won't do you any good to look back and say, "I should have or I could have done this or that." At that moment in time, you did not have the experience to come to another decision.

A mother recently told me that she loved her kids so much that she spent hours explaining the world to them. Everything they did, everywhere they went, whatever they saw, was explained to them. She saw this investment of time and energy as the ultimate expression of love. She wanted her kids to be super intelligent.

When I asked her to see the drawbacks of her love, she could not find any. So I pointed her into a new direction she had probably never thought about before.

You gave your lopsided version of the truth. You ignored and neglected their fantasy. You filled their minds with preselected answers and reduced their ability to think outside of the box. You were probably a nuisance. When others just enjoyed the moment, you had to reduce this magnificent world to words and explanations. Do your kids resent you for being their constant teacher?

When I looked at her, I could see I had hit a nerve. When I asked if her kids had ever asked her to stop with her explanations and just be, she nodded and started to cry. The reason she attended the workshop was because her kids did not allow the grandchildren to stay with her so she could not fill their heads with her version of the truth, which was, as it turned out, very fanatically religious.

Anything good is equally bad.

Believe me, there is no way you can do something that is perceived only good or only bad. It's always both. Having two sides to every issue creates balance.

☯ THE TYRANT AND THE OPPRESSED

If you feel disempowered and self-minimized, and you look up to others (envy, jealousy, admiration, obedience), they have no other choice but to look down on you. It's the natural response. Depending on the intensity of the imbalance, they will treat you accordingly. Guru and disciple, master and slave, boss and employee, tyrant and oppressed; they actually balance each other out. They attract each other like magnets.

If you are disempowered in only ONE area of life and others look down on you, then that's a pain, but it can easily be mended if you focus your attention towards resolving the issue. Learning to resolve the problem is easy.

But if you have three or more areas, which need to be challenged by your loved ones and partners, it's obviously a very stressful situation. Life becomes overwhelming. You are in a constant battle, which is very exhausting. You have little to no chance to live out your dreams; therefore, you tend to feel stressed. Eighty percent of the world population falls into this category.

People who are disempowered in more than four areas of life tend to attract a massive bully. It's almost as cruel as in nature where the weakest is banished from the herd. If they are not fit for survival, they will be teased, bullied and even physically hurt or killed.

It is common for women, who have no financial income, no career, no recognition, no education, no purpose (other than serving their family), no physical passion for sports and well-being, to have serious bullies at home. It might be in the form of a husband, children, parents or all of them together.

It's like a stool with one leg; it falls over easily. Two legs are also unstable and will topple over, attracting criticism and bullies. With three legs, the stool is partially stable and can remain upright and the bullying will reduce. With four legs, the stool stands solid and stable.

Many of my female clients, who had been bullied and beaten by their partner, changed their situation simply by getting a job and earning money; through that they obtained self-respect. Because of the job, they began to care more about their appearance.

The result was that all of their partners changed or vanished. They had fulfilled their job. There was no need to balance anything anymore. Once she made changes in herself, the bully relaxed or disappeared.

If you look at countries with a dictator or a dictatorial regime, you will always find that the population is disempowered.

Let's take the USA as an example. The American people are in financial ruin, with mortgages way over budget, there is no economic growth and, therefore, no jobs to be found, education is at an all-time low, social recognition has been devastated, physical health is deteriorating beyond a measurable or manageable scale, and family values are collapsing as well.

No wonder they attract bullies like the pharmaceutical industry and large corporations, who destroy the last bit of self-value there is left. No wonder these people are mass medicated and force-fed with food, which makes them sick.

As long as the population of the United States does not empower themselves with better education, better health, more passion and self-esteem, a sound purpose and good relationship with each other, they will not find peace.

And you can see that's what is happening.

Education comes over the Internet, demonstrations and rebellion sweeps the country. Communities' gather and share important information, and empowerment is on the way. The Internet is the main tool of the rebellion.

The bully is not the bad guy. He just shows the weakness of those being bullied.

If it were not for the bully, the weak would never have a reason to stand up and would remain in a state of disempowerment, deprivation and devastation.

☯ THE PURPOSE OF LIFE

As a final chapter, I thought I would share with you an image, which has changed my life, and the lives of many of my students. It's a visualization of YOU in all your different forms of energy.

If you would like to learn more about this image, please go to www. EQacademy.com into the members' area and watch a video where I explain the concept in more detail.

This image describes your journey through evolution, your purpose and your present state of mind. This image incorporates every religious belief structure I have studied over the years. In fact, it's a culmination of all the different religions drawn into this one image. You will find many expressions and names of the same thing united into a simple concept.

This image is what I call beyond religion. It is a description of our spiritual journey to what many call GOD.

In relationship to health, I believe this is one of the most important subjects a patient, or in fact any person, should study, as we all have to face the fact that we all have to go one day. No one lives beyond the age of approximately 120 and therefore it's essential to understand:

- Where do we go?
- What comes thereafter?

- Where does this immense amount of compressed energy go, which fires every cell and atomic structure of our being?
- Does it evaporate?
- What is our purpose?
- What have we achieved?
- Who is right?
- Those who think this was a once and only trip or those who say we come back?
- If we come back, what will return?
- How will my next life be?
- Do I have a choice?

These were the questions which fired my research and studies for many years, until I found this answer.

What remains is what the ancients called the individual soul. It's the condensed accumulation of all your memories and beliefs. It's how you remember yourself to be.

> *Energy is never lost or gained. It just transforms from one form to another. Which means, if you die, your energy is not lost but transformed.*

But let's start properly from the beginning.

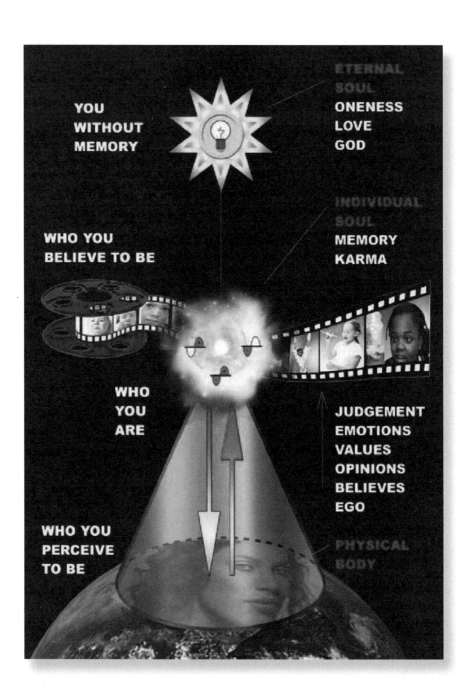

- **The Black Background**

The black background of the image could be described as the container in which everything unfolds. This quantum space is beyond matter. It's what the ancients called akasha, ether, etheric space, the void, infinity, God, Brahma, nirvana and paradise. Throughout history, there have been many names for this oneness.

This space is completely unconditioned. It's the birthplace of all things. Max Planck gave this space a name and dimension by defining the quantum or 1 Planck's dimension.

Modern science has calculated the frequency of this realm as 10-35m to define the so-called starting point of the quantum theory.

- **Eternal Soul**

The light on top of the image represents the eternal life force. It represents God in a more concentrated form than the quantum space. This light animates everything there is with energy. It's without judgment, beliefs and memory. Just like the sun shines without discrimination so does this light radiate energy to each of us.

Once you unite with this energy, you are completely liberated. It's when you become one with everything. Jesus, Buddha, Brahma are known to have reached this state. They have reunited with God. They have returned to paradise. They have dissolved all their beliefs and charges and have no reason/karma to return.

This light is called the eternal soul or the all-pervading soul with infinite potentiality. It is the life energy, which animates everything there is.

The light (thin line) which radiates from this eternal soul is called life spark or life energy and was named in different religions as the Holy Spirit, the breath of Brahma, or OM, the eternal sound.

This pure white light / sound is invisible and unpolarized in space. Only when it meets an object is it reflected, polarized and visible. This is where energy becomes visible as matter.

Just like light which travels from the sun to earth is invisible in space so is this form of energy invisible. When it's polarized and reflected from condensed energy, it takes on the color of the thought.

- **Individual Soul**

The golden cloud with the charged quantum curves in the center of the picture represents YOUR individual soul **with memory**. The more charged memory, the thicker and denser the cloud. This cloud has many names. Some call it EGO, as it feels separate from the all-pervading oneness. It is also called the subconscious or unconscious mind, as it holds your karma, memories, habits and emotional charges. This individual soul is like a memory bank or hard drive in space, which stores your beliefs and charges. This soul has no capability on its own to process or edit the stored information. The cloud needs the body and our worldly experience to actually intensify the charge or to dissolve it.

In case you believe in reincarnation, then this cloud would contain all the thoughts and all the charged memories you ever had from all your previous and your present life. If you prefer to stick only to your present life, then it would contain all of your programming from conception to NOW.

This cloud fulfills two purposes, indicated by the two arrows in opposite directions.

The OBSERVER, as every experience on earth is observed and each memory and beliefs is stored in the subconscious cloud. (We have clarified earlier that memory is always charged).

The other function is what I have represented as the filmstrip. It projects what is stored in your subconscious mind onto the surface of the earth, where you see the movie of your charged thoughts and beliefs unfold.

The movie you watch is based on your emotional charges. If you believe in fairies, you will see them. If you believe in monsters, you will see them. The same is valid for success, health, fame and loving relationships. Whatever is stored in the cloud will be projected into your life. You see what you recognize. The rest is and will be invisible to you. (Remember the filter of beliefs in the fishbowl on your head?)

I've just remembered another example, which describes the filter very well. If you have problems writing without grammatical and spelling errors, you can read the same document 20 times, you will not see what's wrong. Someone who on the other side has learned and mastered this field will go over the same document and find hundreds of errors. We all recognize what we know. Anything else is lost in space.

The cloud can be described in the following way.

- Loads of charges = dark heavy rain cloud with thunder and lightning.

- People who are known to be fanatic and obsessed with beliefs that their way is the only one have a very hard time and in general a huge opposition. Their life resembles often a drama with very little light.

- Little charges = light white fluffy cloud high above the ground.

- Those who have learned to see life from an emotionally intelligent perspective do not need to defend their beliefs, as they know there's not only one way of seeing the world and it would be boring if there were not others with different viewpoints. This attitude is very light and easy to live with. It's actually very refreshing to meet someone who has this status. Due to the fact that these people are not bound to react in a particular way, dictated by their beliefs, they see far more opportunities.

- No charge = no cloud. This is the state where you actually realize peace, stillness, love and oneness with God.

I have met a few people who work very diligently on this kind of non-judgment. They usually live quite secluded and dedicate their life to meditation and a form of prayer which stills the chatter of the mind. All of them hold very powerful positions and are very influential. I attribute this power to what they have achieved in their personal evolution, as all of them have empowered all areas of life equally. They radiate a kind of peace and authority which is hard to describe.

Coming back to the image.

The memory, which is visualized in the form of a movie, projects all of your charged opinions onto the earth. It reflects your EGO and your consciousness. This cloud represents your destiny, karma, talents, abilities, values and preferences, your emotional charges and your subconscious memory.

The individual soul has a **HIGHER MIND**, through which you connect with this eternal soul. This higher mind is called astral body, quantum body or spiritual body.

The medium through which you communicate with the eternal soul is intuition, inspiration, and purpose. The instrument through which you connect is SILENCE. You need to silence the chatter of the mind in order to be able to connect with the eternal soul. You need to practice non-judgment, emotional intelligence and meditation. They are the main tools to tap into the unlimited source of potentiality.

The individual soul also has a **LOWER MIND**, through which we connect to our physical body. This lower mind is usually called emotional body or vibrational body, which connects to the body via instinct, impulse, passion, judgment, opinion, belief and separation.

Every time you reconfirm a particular charge, you confirm a lopsided imprint into the subconscious mind and through that separate yourself even further from the light.

- **Physical Body**

Who you perceive yourself to be. This is our mortal self, dust to dust.

Our physical body and all of our life circumstances are determined by what we hold in our subconscious mind.

CONCLUSION

Letting go of judgment is not only the fastest way into heaven, but also the fastest way to create heaven on earth. There is no need for war or arguments if you can learn to accept everyone as a fellow traveler on their journey of evolution.

Everybody has their own bowl and is responsible to clear the view by discharging their beliefs. All you can do is to push and balance them so they see where their charges are.

The most powerful effect of seeing the world this way comes with the freedom you gain when you drop away from living your life according to others people's values. It happens as soon as you give yourself permission to be as magnificent as every other flower on the field.

Get connected to our online community at:

www.canceriscurablenow.tv